AN OVERVIEW OF SLEEP APNEA DIAGNOSIS AND TREATMENT in 2024

D. A. Nyberg, BS, JD, PhD

©2024 D.A. Nyberg

This book is dedicated to:

Rosalicia Dolan Torres, MD.

the very best Family Practice OB.

Caring for the marginalized!

This book is dedicated to:

Rosalicia Dolan Torres, MD.

the very best Family Practice OB.

Caring for the marginalized!

AN OVERVIEW OF SLEEP APNEA, DIAGNOSIS AND TREATMENT in 2024

D. A. Nyberg, BS, JD, PhD

PREFACE

As a pastor, perennial student, and someone living with severe sleep apnea, my life has been shaped by a profound understanding of human resilience, both personally and professionally. This book, which delves deeply into sleep apnea—its history, diagnosis, and treatment—is not just a clinical exploration but also a personal journey. As a pastor serving the United Methodist Church, I am committed to fostering hope, community, and healing. This mission extends to every facet of my life, including the battle with a medical condition that, while common, is still deeply misunderstood.

My path as a United Methodist pastor and academic has given me the opportunity to engage with individuals from all walks of life, each with unique challenges, aspirations, and experiences. With degrees in psychology, law, and history, my academic pursuits have further illuminated the intersections between mind, body, and society—perspectives that are crucial in understanding sleep apnea, a condition that transcends simple medical definitions. It affects every aspect of a person's life, from physical health and emotional well-being to relationships and productivity.

Personal Journey with Sleep Apnea

Like many people who are eventually diagnosed with sleep apnea, I was unaware for a long time that this condition was impacting my life. I had always assumed that my feelings of fatigue and lack of rest were byproducts of the busy and often demanding life that comes with being a pastor, teacher, and scholar. Long hours of work, constant engagement with my congregation, and intellectual pursuits can take their toll on anyone's energy levels. For years, I blamed my daytime drowsiness, difficulty concentrating, and frequent headaches on these external factors.

However, the realization that something more serious was at play dawned slowly and painfully. The signs became impossible to ignore. Severe daytime sleepiness turned into a struggle to maintain focus even during the most routine tasks, and nights were marked by chronic restlessness. It was only when my health began to noticeably deteriorate that I sought medical advice. After a long journey of polysomnography (PSG) tests and consultations, I received the diagnosis: severe obstructive sleep apnea.

The diagnosis was both a relief and a revelation. It finally provided an explanation for the years of chronic fatigue, mood fluctuations, and cognitive fog. It also illuminated the serious health risks I faced if I did not take action—high blood pressure, heart disease, and even stroke. Sleep apnea wasn't just affecting my daily functioning; it was threatening my long-term health.

As a pastor, I had always focused on the well-being of others, helping my congregation navigate the spiritual, emotional, and physical challenges they faced. But now, I found myself in a position where I had to confront my own health challenges head-on. The journey of managing and understanding sleep apnea has been one of humility and learning—a journey that, in many ways, parallels my spiritual and academic path. It has compelled me to slow down, reflect, and take deliberate steps to reclaim my health.

Why This Book?

There is no shortage of information about sleep apnea, but I felt there was a need for a comprehensive, yet accessible exploration of this condition—one that integrates scientific research, personal experience, and broader societal insights. As someone trained in psychology, I understand the cognitive and emotional tolls of untreated sleep disorders. My Juris Doctorate has given me a unique perspective on the legal and regulatory challenges related to healthcare access and patient rights, particularly as they pertain to managing chronic conditions like sleep apnea. And my PhD in history provides the lens through which I view sleep apnea as not just a modern medical issue but a condition that has existed across time, affecting people in different ways depending on cultural, technological, and scientific advancements.

This book, therefore, is not merely a guide to understanding sleep apnea, its symptoms, and treatments. It is also an attempt to contextualize the condition within broader societal and personal frameworks. The experience of living with sleep apnea raises important questions about self-awareness, medical advocacy, healthcare policy, and human resilience.

Sleep Apnea Through Different Lenses

My academic background has greatly influenced how I approach the subject matter of this book. Through the lens of psychology, we will explore the cognitive and emotional consequences of untreated sleep apnea. Sleep apnea is far more than just snoring or interrupted sleep—it has deep impacts on mental health, contributing to mood disorders, anxiety, depression, and impaired cognitive function. By understanding how sleep apnea affects the brain and emotions, we can better appreciate the urgency of addressing this condition early and effectively.

As a lawyer, I have been trained to think critically about the rights and responsibilities of both patients and healthcare providers. In the context of sleep apnea, this raises important questions about access to care, insurance coverage, and patient rights. Many individuals with sleep apnea, particularly those from underrepresented or marginalized communities, face systemic barriers to receiving adequate care. Whether it's the cost of diagnostic tests like polysomnography, the financial burden of CPAP machines, or the legalities surrounding insurance coverage, patients often struggle to navigate the complexities of the healthcare system. This book will explore some of these legal and policy challenges, offering insights into how individuals can advocate for themselves within these systems.

From a historical perspective, sleep apnea is a relatively "modern" diagnosis, but its symptoms have likely plagued individuals for centuries, if not millennia. Ancient and medieval medical texts contain descriptions of individuals suffering from what we now recognize as sleep-disordered breathing. But it wasn't until the latter half of the 20th century that sleep apnea was formally identified and treated. The history of sleep apnea treatment—from early understandings of snoring to the development of CPAP machines and surgical options—is a fascinating journey of medical innovation. By understanding the historical context of sleep disorders, we can appreciate how far we've come and what the future might hold in terms of treatment advancements.

awareness, medical advocacy, healthcare policy, and human resilience.

Sleep Apnea Through Different Lenses

My academic background has greatly influenced how I approach the subject matter of this book. Through the lens of psychology, we will explore the cognitive and emotional consequences of untreated sleep apnea. Sleep apnea is far more than just snoring or interrupted sleep—it has deep impacts on mental health, contributing to mood disorders, anxiety, depression, and impaired cognitive function. By understanding how sleep apnea affects the brain and emotions, we can better appreciate the urgency of addressing this condition early and effectively.

As a lawyer, I have been trained to think critically about the rights and responsibilities of both patients and healthcare providers. In the context of sleep apnea, this raises important questions about access to care, insurance coverage, and patient rights. Many individuals with sleep apnea, particularly those from underrepresented or marginalized communities, face systemic barriers to receiving adequate care. Whether it's the cost of diagnostic tests like polysomnography, the financial burden of CPAP machines, or the legalities surrounding insurance coverage, patients often struggle to navigate the complexities of the healthcare system. This book will explore some of these legal and policy challenges, offering insights into how individuals can advocate for themselves within these systems.

From a historical perspective, sleep apnea is a relatively "modern" diagnosis, but its symptoms have likely plagued individuals for centuries, if not millennia. Ancient and medieval medical texts contain descriptions of individuals suffering from what we now recognize as sleep-disordered breathing. But it wasn't until the latter half of the 20th century that sleep apnea was formally identified and treated. The history of sleep apnea treatment—from early understandings of snoring to the development of CPAP machines and surgical options—is a fascinating journey of medical innovation. By understanding the historical context of sleep disorders, we can appreciate how far we've come and what the future might hold in terms of treatment advancements.

Spirituality and Health

As a pastor, I am acutely aware of the interconnectedness of spirituality and health. Sleep apnea, like any chronic illness, can be deeply isolating and can challenge one's sense of well-being and purpose. Many of my parishioners have come to me over the years struggling with their own health issues, and I have witnessed firsthand how illness can cause individuals to question their faith, lose hope, or feel disconnected from their spiritual communities.

Living with sleep apnea has deepened my understanding of these struggles, and it has reinforced the importance of compassionate care—both for oneself and others. Self-care is a spiritual practice in its own right, and learning to manage sleep apnea has been an exercise in patience, acceptance, and resilience. Just as we seek spiritual healing through prayer, reflection, and connection with our communities, we must also seek physical healing through medical treatment, lifestyle changes, and self-advocacy.

I encourage you to explore the spiritual dimensions of living with a chronic condition. Faith, hope, and healing are central to human experience, and they play a significant role in how we cope with illness. Sleep apnea, in its own way, can be a reminder of the fragility of the human body and the importance of rest, both physical and spiritual. Learning to live with and manage sleep apnea has been a personal journey of reconciling the demands of a busy life with the need for deep, restorative sleep.

For many people, particularly those in leadership or caregiving roles, there is an expectation to constantly be available—to serve, to provide support for others. But sleep apnea has taught me the importance of setting boundaries and taking time for oneself. Rest is not a luxury; it is a necessity. It is only through rest—both physical and spiritual—that we can continue to do the work we are called to do.

A Call to Action

This book is not just a clinical examination of sleep apnea—it is also a call to action for anyone living with this condition or supporting someone who is. Sleep apnea is a serious and often underdiagnosed disorder, but it is also treatable. Early diagnosis and intervention can prevent many of the long-term health complications associated with untreated sleep apnea. Whether it's through lifestyle changes, PAP therapy, surgery, or emerging treatments, there are options available to help individuals manage their condition and improve their quality of life.

For those in leadership positions, whether in spiritual communities, workplaces, or homes, I urge you to model self-care and encourage those around you to seek help if they suspect they have sleep apnea or any other health condition. By raising awareness, advocating for better access to treatment, and supporting those who are struggling, we can reduce the stigma surrounding sleep disorders and ensure that more individuals receive the care they need.

For healthcare professionals, it is essential to recognize the individualized nature of sleep apnea. No two patients are alike, and effective treatment requires a personalized approach that takes into account a patient's medical history, lifestyle, and preferences. Education and ongoing support are critical to helping patients adhere to their treatment plans and manage the challenges of living with sleep apnea.

And finally, for anyone living with sleep apnea, know that you are not alone. Managing sleep apnea can be challenging, but it is possible to lead a healthy, fulfilling life with the right treatment and support. Whether you are just beginning your journey or have been living with sleep apnea for years, this book is here to provide the information, insights, and encouragement you need to take control of your health.

Conclusion

This preface serves as both an introduction to the content of this book and a personal reflection on my experiences as a pastor, scholar, and individual living with sleep apnea. It is my hope that the information contained within these pages will not only inform but also inspire. Sleep apnea may be a complex and sometimes frustrating condition, but with the right knowledge, support, and treatment, it is possible to reclaim your health and live a life filled with energy, purpose, and peace. As you embark on your own journey—whether as a patient, caregiver, or healthcare provider—I invite you to join me in exploring the many facets of sleep apnea and discovering the ways we can all contribute to a future where this condition is better understood, treated, and managed.

TABLE OF CONTENTS

Introduction --- 27

Overview of Sleep Apnea: ---27

> Define sleep apnea, describe its importance as a public health issue, and provide statistics on prevalence and impact.

Purpose of the Book: ---29

> Explain the aim of providing a comprehensive understanding of the disorder, covering history, diagnosis, treatment options, and challenges.

Structure of the Book: ---31

> Outline the chapters and how they will progress from history and diagnostics to treatment approaches and complexities in managing the condition.

Chapter 1: History of Sleep Apnea --- 37

Early Understanding and Misconceptions: ---37

> Describe early notions of sleep-disordered breathing in ancient and medieval times, focusing on snoring.

First Clinical Descriptions: ---38

> In-depth review of Dr. Gastaut's first clinical descriptions in the 1960s and the development of the apnea concept.

Development of CPAP: ---40

> Dr. Colin Sullivan's invention of CPAP in 1981 as the revolutionary treatment for OSA.

Milestones in Diagnosis and Treatment: ---42

> The evolution of diagnostic technology (e.g., polysomnography) and the introduction of other PAP therapies.

Current Understanding: ---44

> Overview of sleep apnea's relationship with cardiovascular diseases, metabolic syndromes, and the modern view of its broader health risks.

Chapter 2: Types of Sleep Apnea ---49

Obstructive Sleep Apnea (OSA): ---50

> Define and explain the mechanisms behind OSA, including the collapse of the upper airway.

Central Sleep Apnea (CSA): ---56

> Define and explain how the brain fails to signal proper breathing, leading to CSA.

Complex Sleep Apnea: ---60

> Explain the hybrid form that combines OSA and CSA, often seen in patients treated with PAP devices.

Comparison of Types: ---63

> Discuss how these different types present distinct diagnostic challenges and require different treatments.

Chapter 3: Diagnostic Methods in Sleep Apnea 65

Polysomnography (PSG): ---66

> Describe the "gold standard" sleep study, covering the technology used, parameters measured, and interpretation of results.
>
> Explain indices like AHI (Apnea-Hypopnea Index) and ODI (Oxygen Desaturation Index).

Home Sleep Apnea Testing (HSAT): ---71

> Detail the benefits and limitations of portable home tests compared to PSG.
>
> Review typical devices used and their effectiveness in diagnosing OSA, focusing on real-world applications.

Peripheral Arterial Tonometry (PAT): ---75

> Explain the science behind PAT technology and its use in newer diagnostic tools.
>
> Define key indices: pAHI (PAT Hypopnea Index), pRDI (PAT Respiratory Disturbance Index), and their clinical significance.

Oxygenation Measurements: ---78

> Oxygen Saturation (O_2 Sat): Definition and clinical importance in tracking apnea severity.
>
> Mean O_2, Nadir O_2, and Maximum O_2: Detailed explanation of these parameters and their roles in indicating the severity of sleep apnea events.
>
> Oxygen Desaturation Index (ODI): How frequent desaturations (3-4%) are measured and their relevance to risk factors.

Chapter 4: Diagnosis Based on Severity ---83

Mild Sleep Apnea: ---85

>Definition: AHI of 5–14 events/hour.

>Symptoms: Occasional snoring, mild daytime fatigue.

>Diagnostic Signs: Minimal oxygen desaturation (nadir O_2 > 90%), low ODI.

>Consequences of No Treatment: Risks of progression to moderate/severe OSA, increased daytime sleepiness, potential for weight gain.

>Urgency of Treatment: Moderate urgency; lifestyle interventions may suffice initially.

Moderate Sleep Apnea: ---90

>Definition: AHI of 15–29 events/hour.

>Symptoms: Loud snoring, noticeable daytime sleepiness, morning headaches.

>Diagnostic Signs: Moderate oxygen desaturation (nadir O_2 ~85-90%), higher ODI.

Consequences of No Treatment: Higher risk of hypertension, cardiovascular issues, and diminished quality of life.

Urgency of Treatment: High urgency; likely requires CPAP, lifestyle changes, and close monitoring.

Severe Sleep Apnea: ---96

Definition: AHI ≥ 30 events/hour.

Symptoms: Severe daytime sleepiness, choking or gasping during sleep, frequent awakenings.

Diagnostic Signs: Severe oxygen desaturation (nadir O_2 < 85%), very high ODI.

Consequences of No Treatment: Severe cardiovascular risks (stroke, heart attack), high mortality risk.

Urgency of Treatment: Very high urgency; immediate intervention needed with CPAP/BiPAP or surgery.

Chapter 5: Challenges in Diagnosing and Treating Sleep Apnea in Different Body Types ---103

Impact of Body Type on Sleep Apnea: ---104

>Obese Patients: Higher risk of OSA due to airway collapse.

>Thin Patients: More likely to have CSA or complex sleep apnea; challenges in diagnosing and treating severe OSA despite lower body mass.

>Is a Thin Person with Severe Sleep Apnea More Difficult to Treat?

>Diagnostic challenges: Less obvious anatomical causes, more reliance on advanced testing like PSG.

>Treatment approaches: Thin patients may not respond as well to conventional CPAP therapy, requiring advanced devices like BiPAP or ASV.

Chapter 6: Treatment of Mild Sleep Apnea ---123

First-Line Therapies: ---124

>Lifestyle Changes: Weight loss, avoiding alcohol, positional therapy, sleep hygiene improvements.

> Mandibular Advancement Devices (MADs): How they work and when they are indicated.
>
> CPAP for Mild Cases: Lower pressure settings and patient adherence.

Risks of Delaying Treatment: ---138

> Progression to more severe sleep apnea, daytime impairment, and development of comorbidities.

Chapter 7: Treatment Moderate Sleep Apnea 143

PAP Therapy as the Primary Treatment: ---144

> CPAP: First-line therapy, typical settings, and common issues.
>
> BiPAP: Used for patients who struggle with CPAP due to high pressure needs.

Non-PAP Alternatives: ---152

> Mandibular Devices: Effective in moderate cases but with limitations.
>
> Lifestyle Changes: Diet, exercise, and sleep posture interventions.

Consequences of Untreated Moderate OSA: ---158

Risk of cardiovascular complications, hypertension, and reduced life quality.

Chapter 8: Treatment of Severe Sleep Apnea -163

Advanced PAP Therapies: ---164

> BiPAP: Often needed for severe OSA with high pressure requirements.
>
> ASV (Adaptive Servo-Ventilation): Used in patients with complex sleep apnea, adjusting pressures in real-time.
>
> BiPAP Servo-Ventilation: Hybrid approach for those with both central and obstructive events.

Surgical Options: ---173

> UPPP (Uvulopalatopharyngoplasty): Indications, risks, and effectiveness.
>
> Hypoglossal Nerve Stimulation (Inspire Therapy): Emerging treatment for severe OSA.
>
> Other Surgeries: Maxillomandibular advancement, radiofrequency ablation.

Consequences of No Treatment: ---179

High risk of heart attack, stroke, and sudden death.

Chapter 9: New and Emerging Treatment Options ---185

Hypoglossal Nerve Stimulation: ---186

> Mechanism, patient selection, and early outcomes.

Positional Therapy Devices: ---189

> How these devices help reduce apneic events in positional OSA.

Future Directions ---192

Artificial Intelligence in Sleep Apnea Diagnosis and Management: ---192

> AI use to enhance Sleep Studies, Treatment Plans

Current Research in Drug Therapies ---196

> Advances in artificial intelligence for diagnosing and managing sleep apnea, potential drug therapies under research.

Chapter 10: Common Problems in Treatment -201

Adherence to PAP Therapy: ---202

> Common issues: Discomfort, mask leakage, nasal dryness.
>
> Solutions: Mask fitting clinics, humidification, patient education.

Surgical Challenges: ---207

> Variability in outcomes, postoperative complications, and long recovery times.

Insurance and Cost Barriers: ---211

> How cost limits access to advanced treatments.

Chapter 11: The Future of Sleep Apnea Management ---217

Trends in Diagnosis: ---218

> Simplified home tests, wearable technology, and AI.

Innovations in Treatment: ---222

> Advances in PAP technology, personalized medicine, and minimally invasive surgeries.

Innovations in Public Health and Healthcare Policy: ---227

> The need for increased awareness, early screening, and the role of healthcare policy in sleep apnea management.

Conclusion ---233

Recap of Key Points: ---234

> Recap of the most important aspects of diagnosis, treatment, and challenges in managing sleep apnea.

Call to Action: ---238

> Emphasize the importance of early detection, adherence to treatment, and further research to improve patient outcomes.

Bibliography ---243

INTRODUCTION

Overview of Sleep Apnea

Sleep apnea is a common, yet often underdiagnosed sleep disorder characterized by repeated episodes of breathing cessation during sleep. These pauses in breathing, known as apneas, can last from a few seconds to over a minute and can occur multiple times per hour throughout the night. There are three main types of sleep apnea: obstructive sleep apnea (OSA), the most prevalent form; central sleep apnea (CSA), which involves the brain's failure to send proper signals to the muscles that control breathing; and complex sleep apnea, a combination of OSA and CSA.

Obstructive sleep apnea results from the collapse or blockage of the upper airway during sleep, often due to the relaxation of muscles in the throat. In contrast, central sleep apnea stems from a failure in the brain's respiratory control centers. Complex sleep apnea can emerge in patients undergoing treatment for OSA, particularly with positive airway pressure (PAP) therapy.

Sleep apnea is more than a nighttime nuisance. It is a significant public health issue due to its high prevalence and associated health risks, including cardiovascular disease, stroke, diabetes, and impaired cognitive function. According to the American Academy of Sleep Medicine, it is estimated that 29.4 million adults in the United States suffer from OSA, though up to 80% of moderate-to-severe cases remain undiagnosed. Globally, the prevalence varies but is rising due to increasing rates of obesity and aging populations.

The health impact of sleep apnea is profound. Sleep deprivation and intermittent hypoxia, caused by repeated apneas, strain the cardiovascular system and lead to poor sleep quality. Individuals with untreated sleep apnea have a significantly increased risk of hypertension, heart failure, atrial fibrillation, and stroke. Additionally, the disorder negatively affects daytime functioning, contributing to excessive daytime sleepiness, impaired cognitive performance, and mood disorders like depression and anxiety. This combination of risks underscores the importance of recognizing sleep apnea as a serious medical condition that requires early detection and effective treatment.

Purpose of the Book

The purpose of this book is to provide a comprehensive understanding of sleep apnea, drawing from a wide body of medical research and clinical experiences. Sleep apnea has only gained mainstream recognition in the last few decades, and this book aims to bridge the gap between scientific knowledge and public awareness. By exploring the history, diagnostic advancements, treatment innovations, and ongoing challenges, this book will serve as a resource for healthcare professionals, patients, and anyone interested in sleep health.

This book seeks to achieve three primary goals:

1. Educate readers on the history and evolution of sleep apnea: From the earliest misinterpretations of snoring and disordered breathing to the modern understanding of the condition, this book will trace the development of sleep apnea as a distinct medical disorder.

2. Present the latest advancements in diagnosis and treatment: A wide range of diagnostic tools

and therapies are now available for managing sleep apnea, but the choice of treatment depends on several factors, including the type and severity of the disorder. Readers will gain insights into both gold-standard treatments like continuous positive airway pressure (CPAP) therapy and newer innovations such as hypoglossal nerve stimulation.

3. Address challenges in managing sleep apnea: Despite advancements in treatment, many patients continue to struggle with adherence to therapies or experience unresolved symptoms. This book will examine these challenges, from body-type-specific treatment difficulties to issues related to costs and access to care, offering a holistic view of the disorder's complexities.

By the end of the book, readers should have a clear understanding of the current landscape of sleep apnea diagnosis and treatment, as well as insight into future directions for research and therapy.

Structure of the Book

The book is organized into eleven chapters, each focusing on a specific aspect of sleep apnea, from its historical roots to cutting-edge treatments and future trends. Each chapter builds on the knowledge of the previous one, taking readers from a foundational understanding to a more nuanced grasp of the challenges and innovations in managing the disorder.

Chapter 1: History of Sleep Apnea

This chapter begins with a review of early misconceptions surrounding sleep-disordered breathing, tracing ideas from ancient times to the medical breakthroughs of the 20th century. It will explore the pivotal discoveries that led to the identification of sleep apnea as a clinical condition, including the work of Dr. Henri Gastaut in the 1960s and the invention of CPAP therapy by Dr. Colin Sullivan in 1981.

Chapter 2: Types of Sleep Apnea

This chapter delves into the three primary types of sleep apnea: obstructive sleep apnea, central sleep apnea, and complex sleep apnea. Each type will be explained in detail, including the underlying mechanisms, risk factors, and the distinct challenges each presents in terms of diagnosis and treatment.

Chapter 3: Diagnostic Methods in Sleep Apnea

Here, the book will focus on the various diagnostic tools used to assess sleep apnea, with particular emphasis on polysomnography (PSG), the gold-standard test. Alternatives such as home sleep apnea testing (HSAT) and newer technologies like peripheral arterial tonometry (PAT) will also be discussed. The chapter will explain important metrics like the Apnea-Hypopnea Index (AHI) and Oxygen Desaturation Index (ODI) and their roles in evaluating the severity of sleep apnea.

Chapter 4: Diagnosis Based on Severity

In this chapter, sleep apnea will be classified into mild, moderate, and severe categories, with a discussion of the symptoms, diagnostic markers, and treatment urgency for each level. The consequences of untreated sleep apnea at different severities will also be explored.

Chapter 5: Challenges in Diagnosing and Treating Sleep Apnea in Different Body Types

Body type plays a significant role in the presentation and treatment of sleep apnea. This chapter will explore how obesity increases the risk of OSA, while thin patients often present with more complex cases of CSA or severe OSA. It will also address the challenges in treating patients across different body types.

Chapter 6: Treatment of Mild Sleep Apnea

This chapter focuses on first-line treatments for mild cases of sleep apnea, including lifestyle modifications, mandibular advancement devices (MADs), and CPAP therapy. It will discuss the potential risks of delaying treatment and the benefits of early intervention.

Chapter 7: Treatment of Moderate Sleep Apnea

Moderate sleep apnea often requires more intensive management, typically with PAP therapy. This chapter will explore various treatment modalities, including BiPAP for patients who struggle with CPAP, and non-PAP alternatives like mandibular devices and lifestyle changes.

Chapter 8: Treatment of Severe Sleep Apnea

Patients with severe sleep apnea are at the highest risk for serious health complications. This chapter will cover advanced treatments such as adaptive servo-ventilation (ASV), surgical options like uvulopalatopharyngoplasty (UPPP), and emerging therapies like hypoglossal nerve stimulation.

Chapter 9: New and Emerging Treatment Options

This chapter explores the cutting-edge technologies and future directions in sleep apnea treatment. From positional therapy devices to artificial intelligence (AI)-driven diagnostic tools and potential drug therapies, it will provide a forward-looking perspective on the disorder.

Chapter 10: Common Problems in Treatment

Despite the availability of effective treatments, many patients face difficulties in managing their sleep apnea. This chapter will discuss adherence issues with PAP therapy, surgical complications, and the financial barriers to accessing treatment, providing strategies to overcome these challenges.

Chapter 11: The Future of Sleep Apnea Management

The final chapter will review trends in sleep apnea management, including the role of wearable technologies for diagnosis, advancements in personalized medicine, and the implications of these trends for public health. The chapter will also address the importance of policy changes to improve awareness and access to treatment.

Conclusion

The conclusion will summarize the key points covered in the book, emphasizing the importance of early detection, timely intervention, and adherence to treatment to mitigate the health risks associated with sleep apnea. A call to action will urge patients, healthcare providers, and policymakers to prioritize sleep health and further research into innovative treatments that can improve patient outcomes. Through a deeper understanding of sleep apnea, this book aims to empower readers to take control of their sleep health and improve their quality of life.

CHAPTER 1: HISTORY OF SLEEP APNEA

Early Understanding and Misconceptions

Sleep apnea, as we know it today, has a relatively recent clinical definition, but the concept of disordered breathing during sleep is far older. Snoring, a hallmark of obstructive sleep apnea (OSA), has been mentioned in historical records dating back to ancient civilizations. However, for centuries, snoring was often seen as a benign, if not humorous, characteristic rather than a potential sign of a serious health disorder. This misunderstanding persisted for much of human history, and it is only in the last 50 years that sleep apnea has been recognized as a major medical condition.

In ancient Greece and Rome, snoring was sometimes attributed to indulgence, with excess weight and alcohol consumption being linked to it. However, these ancient texts made little connection between snoring and the more insidious health impacts of sleep-disordered breathing. For instance, Hippocrates, the "father of medicine," alluded to sleep and breathing issues but did not link them to the specific condition we now recognize as sleep apnea. In the medieval period, references to breathing problems during sleep were often couched in terms of religious or superstitious interpretations. Conditions like sleep paralysis were often attributed to demons or spirits pressing on the chest, causing a person to struggle for breath.

It was not until the 19th century that more systematic observations of sleep and breathing began to emerge. Early physicians noted that individuals who snored loudly or struggled to breathe at night often experienced daytime fatigue and a reduced quality of life. In some cases, they even observed that patients would stop breathing altogether for brief periods. Unfortunately, the medical community at the time lacked the tools to fully understand the physiology behind these phenomena, and thus, early studies were largely anecdotal.

First Clinical Descriptions: Dr. Henri Gastaut and the 1960s Breakthrough

The first major leap forward in understanding sleep apnea came in the mid-20th century, specifically in the 1960s, when French neurologist

Dr. Henri Pascal Gastaut (1915-1995) published groundbreaking research on what he termed "obstructive apnea." Gastaut's research provided the first formal clinical descriptions of obstructive sleep apnea, identifying the cyclic cessation of airflow during sleep due to the collapse of the upper airway. This research followed closely on the heels of a broader medical interest in the physiology of sleep, driven by advancements in the study of human consciousness and brain activity.

In a landmark study published in 1965, Gastaut and his colleagues conducted overnight sleep studies on patients with suspected apnea. Using the newly developed technique of polysomnography (PSG), they were able to monitor brain activity, eye movements, muscle tone, heart rate, and breathing patterns simultaneously during sleep. This comprehensive recording method allowed Gastaut to observe that the patients who stopped breathing during sleep often had obstructed airways and collapsed throats, leading to the cessation of airflow despite their continued respiratory effort.

Gastaut's work also drew attention to the fact that obstructive sleep apnea (OSA) was not merely a physical issue but also had serious implications for the cardiovascular and metabolic systems. His research revealed that many of the patients with sleep apnea also had high blood pressure, irregular heartbeats, and other signs of cardiovascular strain. These findings were monumental in shifting the medical perspective on sleep-disordered breathing from a minor inconvenience to a serious health issue.

Around the same time, researchers also began to differentiate central sleep apnea (CSA), in which the brain fails to send proper signals to the muscles that control breathing, from OSA. The work of Gastaut laid the foundation for further exploration of both types of sleep apnea.

Development of CPAP: A Revolution in Sleep Apnea Treatment

Despite the growing awareness of sleep apnea as a distinct medical condition, treatment options remained limited for several years. In the 1970s, most patients diagnosed with sleep apnea were advised to lose weight, avoid alcohol, or undergo tracheostomy, a highly invasive surgical procedure that involved making an incision in the trachea to allow air to bypass the upper airway obstructions. While tracheostomy was effective in relieving airway blockages, it came with significant risks and lifestyle limitations. For many patients, this was not a viable long-term solution.

The breakthrough in treatment came in 1981 with the invention of Continuous Positive Airway Pressure (CPAP) by Australian physician Dr. Colin Edward Sullivan (1945-). Sullivan's invention marked a revolutionary shift in the treatment of obstructive sleep apnea. CPAP therapy involved delivering a continuous stream of air through a mask worn over the nose and mouth, which helped to keep the upper airway open by providing positive pressure. This non-invasive method was immediately effective at preventing airway collapse during sleep, reducing the number of apnea events, and improving sleep quality.

The concept behind CPAP was simple but profoundly impactful. By providing a constant flow of air pressure, the device was able to prevent the tongue and soft tissues in the throat from collapsing and blocking the airway, thus allowing for uninterrupted breathing throughout the night. Dr. Sullivan first tested the device on dogs and later on human subjects with great success. CPAP rapidly became the gold standard for treating obstructive sleep apnea, particularly for moderate to severe cases.

By the mid-1980s, CPAP machines had evolved to become more user-friendly, with various manufacturers producing models that could be adjusted for pressure levels and fitted with different types of masks. The introduction of CPAP therapy not only improved the quality of life for millions of patients but also reduced the long-term risks of untreated sleep apnea, such as cardiovascular disease, stroke, and premature death.

Milestones in Diagnosis and Treatment

The invention of CPAP was followed by significant advances in both the diagnosis and treatment of sleep apnea. The 1980s and 1990s saw the widespread adoption of polysomnography (PSG) in sleep laboratories, allowing physicians to accurately diagnose sleep apnea through overnight studies that measured various physiological parameters during sleep. The Apnea-Hypopnea Index (AHI), which quantifies the severity of sleep apnea based on the number of apnea and hypopnea events per hour of sleep, became the standard metric for diagnosing the disorder.

At the same time, researchers continued to develop alternative treatments for patients who were unable to tolerate CPAP therapy. One of the first alternatives to CPAP was BiPAP (Bilevel Positive Airway Pressure), which provides two levels of air pressure—one for inhalation and another for exhalation. This was particularly helpful for patients with high airway resistance or those who found it difficult to exhale against the continuous pressure of CPAP.

Surgical options also expanded during this period. While tracheostomy remained an option for severe cases, less invasive surgeries, such as uvulopalatopharyngoplasty (UPPP), gained popularity. UPPP involved the removal of excess tissue in the throat, including the uvula and part of the soft palate, to widen the airway. However, the effectiveness of UPPP varied, and the procedure came with risks, including difficulty swallowing and changes in the voice.

In addition to surgical and mechanical treatments, mandibular advancement devices (MADs) were introduced in the 1990s as a treatment for mild to moderate OSA. These oral appliances work by repositioning the lower jaw forward, thereby preventing the collapse of the airway. While effective for certain patients, MADs are generally less effective than CPAP for severe cases of sleep apnea.

Current Understanding of Sleep Apnea

Today, the understanding of sleep apnea has expanded far beyond the early concepts of snoring and disrupted sleep. It is now recognized as a multisystem disorder with widespread health implications. The relationship between sleep apnea and cardiovascular disease is one of the most well-established findings in the field. Numerous studies have shown that individuals with untreated sleep apnea are at significantly higher risk for hypertension, coronary artery disease, heart failure, stroke, and sudden cardiac death.

The mechanisms behind these cardiovascular risks are complex but are thought to involve the intermittent hypoxia (low oxygen levels) and sleep fragmentation that occur with untreated sleep apnea. Repeated drops in blood oxygen levels trigger the sympathetic nervous system, leading to increased heart rate, elevated blood pressure, and inflammation—all of which contribute to long-term cardiovascular damage. Additionally, sleep apnea has been linked to metabolic disorders, including type 2 diabetes and obesity. In fact, the relationship between obesity and sleep apnea is bidirectional: obesity increases the risk of developing OSA, and untreated OSA can contribute to weight gain by disrupting metabolism and increasing insulin resistance.

In the last two decades, researchers have also uncovered links between sleep apnea and cognitive decline, particularly in older adults. Chronic sleep disruption and intermittent hypoxia may contribute to neurodegenerative diseases such as Alzheimer's disease, as well as impairments in memory, attention, and executive function. Furthermore, sleep apnea has been associated with mental health disorders such as depression and anxiety, likely due to the impact of poor sleep quality on mood regulation.

The current understanding of sleep apnea has also expanded to recognize its prevalence in children and adolescents, who may present with different symptoms compared to adults. In children, sleep apnea is often related to enlarged tonsils and adenoids and may manifest as hyperactivity, behavioral problems, or difficulty concentrating rather than the classic symptoms of snoring and daytime sleepiness. Untreated pediatric sleep apnea can lead to developmental and learning difficulties, highlighting the importance of early diagnosis and treatment.

With advancements in technology, home sleep apnea testing (HSAT) has become a valuable tool for diagnosing OSA in patients who cannot or do not wish to undergo an overnight sleep study in a lab. While not as comprehensive as polysomnography, HSAT devices can measure airflow, respiratory effort, and oxygen levels, making them a convenient and cost-effective option for diagnosing moderate to severe sleep apnea in appropriate patients.

Conclusion

The history of sleep apnea reflects a journey from early misconceptions and anecdotal observations to a sophisticated understanding of a multisystem disorder with profound implications for health. From the first clinical descriptions by Dr. Henri Gastaut in the 1960s to the revolutionary development of CPAP by Dr. Colin Sullivan in 1981, the medical community has made enormous strides in diagnosing and treating sleep apnea. Today, with advanced diagnostic tools, a range of therapeutic options, and ongoing research into the connections between sleep apnea and other health conditions, sleep medicine continues to evolve, offering hope for millions of individuals affected by this condition.

Sleep apnea has gone from a poorly understood phenomenon to a well-recognized public health concern. The knowledge gained over the last 50 years has laid a strong foundation for the future, but challenges remain, particularly in ensuring early diagnosis, patient adherence to treatment, and access to care for all who need it. As research continues to explore new frontiers, from artificial intelligence in diagnostics to novel therapies like hypoglossal nerve stimulation, the outlook for patients with sleep apnea is promising.

CHAPTER 2: TYPES OF SLEEP APNEA

Introduction

Sleep apnea is broadly categorized into three main types: Obstructive Sleep Apnea (OSA), Central Sleep Apnea (CSA), and Complex Sleep Apnea Syndrome (CompSAS), also referred to as treatment-emergent central sleep apnea. These types differ in their causes, mechanisms, symptoms, and treatment approaches. However, they share a common feature—interrupted breathing during sleep, leading to poor sleep quality and serious health risks.

Understanding the different types of sleep apnea is essential for proper diagnosis and management, as each type requires specific treatment strategies. In this chapter, we will explore the mechanisms, clinical presentations, diagnostic challenges, and treatment options for each type of sleep apnea, followed by a comparison of their key differences and overlaps.

Obstructive Sleep Apnea (OSA)

Obstructive Sleep Apnea (OSA) is by far the most common type of sleep apnea, accounting for approximately 84% of all cases. OSA occurs when the muscles in the back of the throat relax excessively during sleep, causing a temporary collapse or blockage of the upper airway. This leads to repeated interruptions in breathing, known as apneas, and subsequent drops in blood oxygen levels.

Mechanism Behind OSA

OSA is primarily caused by the anatomical structure of the upper airway and the physiological behavior of the muscles involved in breathing. During normal sleep, the muscles in the throat relax, but in individuals with OSA, this relaxation is exaggerated, leading to airway obstruction. This obstruction is often exacerbated by additional factors such as obesity, large tonsils, a receded chin, or other anatomical abnormalities that narrow the airway. When the airway is blocked, the diaphragm and chest muscles work harder to pull air into the lungs, but the effort is often unsuccessful until the brain detects the lack of oxygen and briefly awakens the individual to reopen the airway. This momentary awakening, known as an arousal, is often so brief that the person is unaware of it, though it severely disrupts sleep.

Once the individual briefly wakes up, the muscles tighten, the airway opens, and normal breathing resumes, often accompanied by a snorting or gasping sound. This cycle can repeat anywhere from five to over a hundred times per hour, leading to fragmented, non-restorative sleep. In addition to the direct effects of disrupted breathing, individuals with OSA often experience hypopneas (shallow breathing episodes) that reduce airflow but do not completely block it.

Symptoms and Clinical Presentation

The symptoms of OSA can be divided into nocturnal (occurring during sleep) and daytime symptoms. Nocturnal symptoms are often first noticed by a bed partner and include:

Loud, chronic snoring: Snoring is a hallmark feature of OSA, caused by the vibration of tissues in the throat as air struggles to pass through a narrowed airway.

Gasping or choking during sleep: Bed partners may report witnessing the individual stop breathing, followed by loud gasps or choking sounds.

Frequent awakenings: Although individuals with OSA may not remember waking up during the night, they often experience multiple arousals due to apneas and hypopneas.

Frequent urination (nocturia): Some people with OSA wake up multiple times during the night to urinate, a symptom likely linked to the body's response to oxygen deprivation.

Daytime symptoms include:

Excessive daytime sleepiness: This is one of the most common complaints from individuals with OSA, caused by fragmented sleep and poor sleep quality.

Morning headaches: Repeated episodes of low oxygen levels can cause vascular changes in the brain, leading to headaches.

Difficulty concentrating and memory problems: Cognitive function can be impaired due to chronic sleep deprivation.

Mood disturbances: Depression, irritability, and anxiety are common in individuals with untreated OSA.

Dry mouth or sore throat: Some people wake up with a dry mouth or sore throat due to mouth breathing during apneas.

Risk Factors for OSA

Certain factors increase the likelihood of developing OSA, including:

Obesity: The most significant risk factor for OSA, with increased fat deposits around the neck narrowing the airway.

Male gender: OSA is more common in men than women, although postmenopausal women have a higher risk.

Age: The risk of OSA increases with age, particularly after 50.

Family history: Genetic factors play a role in the anatomical characteristics that predispose individuals to OSA.

Alcohol and sedative use: These substances relax the muscles in the throat, increasing the risk of airway collapse.

Smoking: Smoking can cause inflammation and fluid retention in the upper airway, exacerbating the risk of obstruction.

Diagnosis of OSA

OSA is typically diagnosed through polysomnography (PSG), an overnight sleep study that measures multiple physiological parameters, including airflow, oxygen levels, and brain activity. The Apnea-Hypopnea Index (AHI), which counts the number of apneas and hypopneas per hour, is used to assess the severity of OSA:

> Mild OSA: 5–14 events per hour
>
> Moderate OSA: 15–29 events per hour
>
> Severe OSA: 30 or more events per hour

In some cases, home sleep apnea testing (HSAT) may be used for diagnosis, though it is less comprehensive than in-lab polysomnography.

Treatment of OSA

The first-line treatment for OSA is Continuous Positive Airway Pressure (CPAP) therapy, which involves wearing a mask connected to a machine that delivers a continuous stream of air to keep the airway open during sleep. CPAP is highly effective but can be difficult for some patients to tolerate. Other treatments include:

Mandibular Advancement Devices (MADs): Oral appliances that reposition the lower jaw to prevent airway collapse, used for mild to moderate cases.

Positional therapy: Recommended for patients whose OSA is worse when sleeping on their back.

Weight loss: Losing weight can significantly reduce the severity of OSA in overweight individuals.

Surgical options: In cases where CPAP or MADs are ineffective, surgery to remove excess tissue (such as uvulopalatopharyngoplasty) or reposition the jaw may be considered.

Central Sleep Apnea (CSA)

Central Sleep Apnea (CSA) is less common than OSA, accounting for approximately 5-10% of all sleep apnea cases. CSA occurs when the brain fails to send appropriate signals to the muscles that control breathing. Unlike OSA, where airway obstruction is the primary issue, CSA is characterized by repeated pauses in breathing due to a lack of respiratory effort.

Mechanism Behind CSA

In CSA, the problem lies in the brain's respiratory control centers located in the brainstem. These centers regulate the rate and depth of breathing by responding to changes in carbon dioxide (CO_2) and oxygen levels in the blood. In individuals with CSA, the brain does not respond appropriately to changes in CO_2 and oxygen, leading to periodic pauses in breathing. Unlike OSA, where the airway collapses, the airway remains open in CSA, but breathing stops because the muscles that control respiration are not activated.

There are several subtypes of CSA, including:

Cheyne-Stokes respiration: A pattern of waxing and waning breathing, often seen in patients with heart failure or stroke.

Idiopathic CSA: CSA without a known cause.

CSA due to medical conditions: Such as heart failure, stroke, or high-altitude exposure.

CSA due to opioid use: Long-term use of opioids can suppress the brain's ability to regulate breathing.

Symptoms and Clinical Presentation

The symptoms of CSA overlap with those of OSA but may be less obvious, as CSA is less likely to cause loud snoring. The main symptoms include:

Periodic breathing: Pauses in breathing that may be followed by deep, rapid breaths.

Frequent awakenings during the night: Often without a clear cause.

Daytime fatigue: Due to disrupted sleep.

Morning headaches: Likely due to reduced oxygen levels during the night.

Difficulty staying asleep (insomnia): Many individuals with CSA report frequent awakenings throughout the night.

Risk Factors for CSA

Several factors can increase the risk of developing CSA, including:

Heart failure: CSA is common in individuals with congestive heart failure, particularly those with Cheyne-Stokes breathing.

Stroke: A stroke affecting the brainstem can impair the respiratory control centers, leading to CSA.

Chronic opioid use: Long-term use of opioids can depress the respiratory system and cause CSA.

High-altitude exposure: Living or traveling to high altitudes, where oxygen levels are lower, can trigger CSA.

Diagnosis of CSA

Like OSA, CSA is diagnosed using polysomnography. The key difference in the diagnosis of CSA is that the absence of airflow is accompanied by a lack of respiratory effort, which can be detected by monitoring the movement of the chest and abdomen during sleep. The Apnea-Hypopnea Index (AHI) is also used to classify the severity of CSA, though it may be accompanied by additional measurements of heart and brain function in patients with underlying conditions like heart failure.

Treatment of CSA

Treatment for CSA depends on the underlying cause. In some cases, treating the underlying condition, such as heart failure, can reduce or eliminate CSA. Specific treatment options for CSA include:

Adaptive Servo-Ventilation (ASV): A type of positive airway pressure (PAP) therapy designed specifically for CSA, which adjusts the pressure delivered during each breath to maintain normal breathing patterns.

Bi-level Positive Airway Pressure (BiPAP): Provides two levels of pressure—one for inhalation and another for exhalation. It is used in some cases of CSA, particularly for patients with central apnea due to neuromuscular diseases.

Medications: Such as acetazolamide or theophylline, which stimulate breathing by altering the body's response to CO_2 levels.

Oxygen therapy: In some cases, supplemental oxygen may be used to prevent drops in blood oxygen levels during sleep.

Complex Sleep Apnea (CompSAS)

Complex Sleep Apnea Syndrome (CompSAS), also known as treatment-emergent central sleep apnea, is a relatively new classification. It occurs when patients who are being treated for OSA with PAP therapy begin to develop central apneas during treatment. Initially, these patients present with OSA, but after starting PAP therapy, central apneas emerge, leading to a combination of obstructive and central events.

Mechanism Behind CompSAS

The precise mechanism of CompSAS is not fully understood, but it is thought to involve a disruption in the body's respiratory control mechanisms caused by the use of PAP therapy. The increased pressure from PAP may reduce CO_2 levels in the blood, leading to a failure of the brain's respiratory centers to trigger breathing. This condition is particularly perplexing because the patient appears to have resolved the obstructive component of their apnea, only to develop central apneas.

Symptoms and Clinical Presentation

Patients with CompSAS often present with a combination of OSA and CSA symptoms, including:

Persistent apneas despite the use of PAP therapy.

Symptoms of poor sleep quality, such as daytime fatigue, frequent awakenings, and difficulty concentrating.

Mixed episodes of snoring and periods of silence during sleep.

Risk Factors for CompSAS

Use of CPAP or BiPAP: CompSAS is typically diagnosed in patients who begin treatment for OSA with PAP therapy and develop central apneas.

Heart failure: Like CSA, patients with heart failure are at higher risk for developing CompSAS.

Neuromuscular diseases: Conditions that affect the respiratory muscles can increase the risk of developing central apneas.

Diagnosis of CompSAS

Diagnosis of CompSAS is challenging because it requires distinguishing between obstructive and central events, both of which can occur simultaneously in patients. Polysomnography with PAP therapy in place is the standard diagnostic tool, allowing for the detection of central apneas that emerge during treatment.

Treatment of CompSAS

The treatment of CompSAS can be complex, as standard CPAP therapy may exacerbate the central apneas. Adaptive Servo-Ventilation (ASV) is often the treatment of choice for patients with CompSAS, as it adjusts the pressure delivered during each breath based on the patient's breathing patterns, thereby preventing central apneas. In some cases, adjusting the settings on the patient's existing PAP device may resolve the issue, while others may require oxygen therapy or medications to stabilize breathing.

Comparison of Types

While OSA, CSA, and CompSAS share the feature of interrupted breathing during sleep, the underlying mechanisms and treatments differ significantly. OSA is primarily a mechanical issue, involving the collapse of the upper airway, while CSA is a neurological condition where the brain fails to signal the need for breathing. CompSAS adds another layer of complexity by involving a combination of both obstructive and central events, typically triggered by the use of PAP therapy.

Diagnosing and treating these conditions requires an understanding of the unique challenges each type presents. For example, OSA is often associated with snoring and excessive daytime sleepiness, while CSA may be harder to detect without the help of specialized sleep studies, as it does not typically cause loud snoring. CompSAS requires clinicians to carefully balance treatments to manage both obstructive and central events, which can be a delicate process.

Conclusion

Understanding the different types of sleep apnea—OSA, CSA, and CompSAS—is crucial for accurate diagnosis and effective treatment. Each type presents unique challenges, and treatment must be tailored to the specific mechanisms behind the disorder. With advancements in diagnostic tools such as polysomnography, home sleep apnea testing, and innovative therapies like ASV, clinicians now have more resources than ever to manage these complex conditions. However, the ongoing challenge remains to ensure that all patients with sleep apnea, regardless of type, receive timely diagnosis and appropriate treatment to improve their quality of life and reduce their risk of serious health complications.

CHAPTER 3: DIAGNOSTIC METHODS IN SLEEP APNEA

Introduction

Diagnosing sleep apnea accurately is critical for determining the appropriate treatment approach and preventing serious complications such as cardiovascular disease, cognitive impairment, and metabolic disorders. Several diagnostic methods are used to assess sleep apnea, ranging from the gold-standard polysomnography (PSG) to less invasive home sleep apnea testing (HSAT) and novel technologies like peripheral arterial tonometry (PAT). The choice of diagnostic method depends on factors such as the severity of symptoms, underlying health conditions, and the resources available to the patient.

This chapter will explore the different diagnostic tools used in sleep apnea assessment, beginning with PSG, followed by home testing options, and newer innovations in diagnostic technology. We will also cover the parameters measured during these tests, such as the Apnea-Hypopnea Index (AHI), Oxygen Desaturation Index (ODI), and various oxygenation measurements, as well as their clinical relevance in diagnosing and assessing the severity of sleep apnea.

Polysomnography (PSG): The Gold Standard

Polysomnography (PSG) is considered the gold standard for diagnosing sleep apnea and other sleep disorders. It is a comprehensive, overnight sleep study that monitors a wide range of physiological parameters during sleep, including brain activity, eye movements, muscle tone, heart rate, respiratory effort, airflow, and blood oxygen levels. By capturing these variables, PSG provides a complete picture of a patient's sleep architecture and the presence of respiratory events such as apneas (cessation of breathing) and hypopneas (reduced airflow).

The Process of Polysomnography

PSG is typically conducted in a sleep laboratory under the supervision of trained sleep technicians. The patient spends a night in the lab while connected to several sensors that record physiological signals. The setup for PSG includes:

Electroencephalography (EEG): Measures brain activity to identify different sleep stages (non-REM and REM sleep) and periods of wakefulness.

Electrooculography (EOG): Tracks eye movements, particularly during REM sleep, when rapid eye movement is most pronounced.

Electromyography (EMG): Measures muscle tone, often focusing on the chin and legs, to detect muscle relaxation and movements.

Electrocardiography (ECG): Monitors heart rate and rhythm, which can reveal cardiovascular strain due to sleep apnea.

Nasal and oral airflow sensors: Measure the rate and volume of airflow through the nose and mouth.

Chest and abdominal belts: Detect respiratory effort by monitoring the expansion and contraction of the chest and abdomen.

Pulse oximetry: Measures oxygen saturation (SpO_2) in the blood, providing information on how well the lungs are oxygenating the blood during sleep.

Microphone: Records snoring and other sounds made during sleep, which can help differentiate between obstructive and central sleep apnea.

PSG Parameters and Their Interpretation

PSG data are analyzed to detect apneas, hypopneas, and other respiratory events. Apneas are defined as complete cessation of airflow for at least 10 seconds, while hypopneas are episodes of reduced airflow that cause a drop in blood oxygen levels. These events are typically categorized as either obstructive (caused by airway collapse), central (caused by a lack of respiratory effort), or mixed (a combination of both).

The following indices are calculated during PSG to assess the severity of sleep apnea:

Apnea-Hypopnea Index (AHI): The AHI is the primary measure of sleep apnea severity, calculated as the average number of apneas and hypopneas per hour of sleep. It is used to classify sleep apnea into three categories:

Mild sleep apnea: 5-14 events per hour

Moderate sleep apnea: 15-29 events per hour

Severe sleep apnea: 30 or more events per hour

A higher AHI indicates more severe sleep apnea and correlates with a greater risk of cardiovascular and metabolic complications.

Oxygen Desaturation Index (ODI): The ODI measures the number of times per hour that blood oxygen levels drop by 3-4% or more during sleep. Repeated episodes of oxygen desaturation are a hallmark of sleep apnea, especially obstructive sleep apnea, and contribute to the long-term health risks associated with the disorder.

Respiratory Disturbance Index (RDI): The RDI includes not only apneas and hypopneas but also respiratory effort-related arousals (RERAs)—events where breathing is partially obstructed, leading to arousal from sleep but not meeting the full criteria for apnea or hypopnea. RERAs can be significant in diagnosing upper airway resistance syndrome (UARS), a condition related to OSA.

Strengths and Limitations of Polysomnography

PSG is the most thorough and reliable method for diagnosing sleep apnea because it captures multiple aspects of sleep and breathing patterns. It provides detailed information about the severity and type of sleep apnea, which is critical for tailoring treatment.

Strengths:

Comprehensive data: PSG monitors multiple physiological variables, allowing for a complete assessment of sleep quality and the identification of other sleep disorders, such as periodic limb movement disorder (PLMD) or narcolepsy.

Accurate differentiation between OSA and CSA: PSG can distinguish between obstructive and central events by measuring respiratory effort.

Highly controlled environment: Conducting the test in a sleep lab ensures that data are collected in a standardized manner with minimal disruptions.

Limitations:

Cost and accessibility: PSG is expensive and not always covered by insurance, making it inaccessible to some patients. It also requires an overnight stay in a sleep lab, which may not be convenient or comfortable for all individuals.

Limited availability: There may be long wait times for PSG, particularly in areas with few sleep labs, delaying diagnosis and treatment.

Artificial sleep environment: Sleeping in a lab with sensors attached to the body may not reflect typical sleep patterns, potentially skewing the results.

Home Sleep Apnea Testing (HSAT)

For patients who may not have access to a sleep lab or for those with high suspicion of moderate to severe OSA, Home Sleep Apnea Testing (HSAT) offers a less invasive, more convenient alternative to in-lab PSG. HSAT devices are portable and designed to be used at home, allowing patients to sleep in their usual environment while recording basic parameters related to sleep apnea.

The Process of HSAT

HSAT typically involves a simplified setup compared to PSG. The devices used for HSAT focus on key parameters related to respiratory events, including:

Airflow: Measured using a nasal cannula or an oral-nasal sensor to detect apneas and hypopneas.

Respiratory effort: Monitored using chest and abdominal belts to detect breathing effort and distinguish between obstructive and central events.

Pulse oximetry: Tracks oxygen saturation levels throughout the night, which is critical for identifying oxygen desaturation events.

Heart rate: Recorded to assess the cardiovascular response to apneas and hypopneas.

Unlike PSG, HSAT does not typically monitor brain activity, eye movements, or muscle tone, meaning it cannot provide detailed information about sleep stages or diagnose other sleep disorders. HSAT is primarily used for diagnosing moderate to severe OSA in patients who have a high pre-test probability based on clinical symptoms.

Benefits and Limitations of HSAT

Benefits:

Convenience and comfort: Patients can perform the test in the comfort of their own home, which may lead to more natural sleep patterns and accurate results.

Cost-effective: HSAT is significantly less expensive than PSG, making it a more affordable option for many patients.

Accessibility: HSAT can be more widely available, particularly in regions where access to sleep labs is limited.

Limitations:

Limited scope: HSAT cannot provide the comprehensive data that PSG offers, making it unsuitable for diagnosing more complex sleep disorders, such as CSA, or conditions involving abnormal sleep architecture.

Accuracy: While HSAT is effective for diagnosing moderate to severe OSA, it may underestimate the severity of the condition or fail to detect mild cases.

Inability to differentiate between OSA and CSA: HSAT does not directly measure respiratory effort, making it difficult to distinguish between obstructive and central apneas without additional testing.

HSAT is typically recommended for patients with a high likelihood of moderate to severe OSA based on clinical evaluation and risk factors. It is less useful for diagnosing CSA, complex sleep apnea, or other sleep-related conditions that require more detailed analysis.

Peripheral Arterial Tonometry (PAT)

In recent years, Peripheral Arterial Tonometry (PAT) has emerged as an innovative, non-invasive method for assessing sleep apnea. PAT measures changes in arterial tone (the constriction and dilation of blood vessels) during sleep, providing indirect evidence of respiratory events. Devices that use PAT technology, such as the WatchPAT, are increasingly being used in both clinical and home settings as an alternative to traditional PSG or HSAT.

Mechanism of PAT

PAT devices use a finger-mounted sensor to detect changes in peripheral arterial tone, which is influenced by the autonomic nervous system. Respiratory events, such as apneas and hypopneas, cause brief arousals from sleep and activate the sympathetic nervous system, leading to vasoconstriction in the blood vessels. By measuring these changes in arterial tone, along with other parameters like pulse oximetry and heart rate,

 PAT devices can estimate the number and severity of respiratory disturbances.

PAT technology measures several key indices:

PAT Apnea-Hypopnea Index (pAHI): Similar to the AHI calculated in PSG, the pAHI reflects the number of apneas and hypopneas per hour of sleep, as estimated by changes in arterial tone and oxygen saturation.

PAT Respiratory Disturbance Index (pRDI): The pRDI includes not only apneas and hypopneas but also more subtle respiratory disturbances that cause arousals, similar to the RDI used in PSG.

True Sleep Time: Unlike traditional HSAT, which may rely on estimates of total sleep time, PAT devices can provide a more accurate measurement of actual sleep time, improving the precision of the pAHI and pRDI calculations.

Benefits and Limitations of PAT

Benefits:

Non-invasive and easy to use: PAT devices are typically more comfortable for patients than traditional sleep study equipment, as they only require a finger-mounted sensor and a few other sensors, making them suitable for home use.

Accurate sleep time estimation: PAT devices can more accurately estimate sleep time than other home testing devices, leading to more reliable indices such as pAHI and pRDI.

Can be used for both OSA and CSA: PAT devices can detect respiratory disturbances caused by both obstructive and central events, making them a versatile tool for diagnosing different types of sleep apnea.

Limitations:

Less comprehensive than PSG: Although PAT provides useful data on respiratory disturbances, it does not offer the same level of detail as PSG, particularly in terms of sleep architecture and brain activity.

Limited availability: While PAT devices are becoming more widely available, they are still less commonly used than traditional PSG or HSAT.

Cost: Although PAT is less expensive than PSG, it may still be more costly than other home testing options, making it less accessible for some patients.

PAT technology is gaining popularity as a middle ground between PSG and HSAT, offering more comprehensive data than traditional home testing devices while being more convenient and accessible than in-lab polysomnography.

Oxygenation Measurements

Oxygen levels during sleep are a critical component of sleep apnea diagnosis and assessment, as apneas and hypopneas can lead to intermittent hypoxia (repeated drops in blood oxygen levels). Several oxygenation parameters are commonly measured during sleep studies, providing insight into the severity of the condition and its potential impact on the patient's health.

Oxygen Saturation (SpO_2)

Oxygen saturation (SpO_2) is the percentage of hemoglobin in the blood that is saturated with oxygen. In healthy individuals, SpO_2 typically remains above 95% during sleep. In patients with sleep apnea, however, repeated apneas and hypopneas can cause significant drops in oxygen levels, leading to hypoxemia. The degree and frequency of these drops are key indicators of the severity of the disorder.

Key Oxygenation Parameters

Several specific oxygenation parameters are used to assess the impact of sleep apnea on blood oxygen levels:

Mean O_2: The average oxygen saturation level throughout the night. A lower mean O_2 suggests that the patient spends a significant portion of the night in a hypoxic state.

Nadir O_2: The lowest oxygen saturation level recorded during the night. A nadir O_2 below 85% is often seen in patients with severe sleep apnea and is associated with a higher risk of cardiovascular and metabolic complications.

Maximum O_2: The highest oxygen saturation level recorded during the night. In healthy individuals, this should remain close to 100%.

Oxygen Desaturation Index (ODI): The ODI measures the number of times per hour that the oxygen saturation drops by 3-4% or more from baseline. A higher ODI indicates more frequent desaturation events, which are linked to increased cardiovascular risk and overall disease burden.

Clinical Relevance of Oxygenation Measurements

Oxygenation measurements are crucial for assessing the severity of sleep apnea and its potential impact on the patient's health. Repeated episodes of hypoxia can lead to oxidative stress, inflammation, and sympathetic nervous system activation, contributing to the development of hypertension, coronary artery disease, stroke, and other serious conditions. Patients with frequent and severe oxygen desaturation are also at higher risk for cognitive impairment and daytime sleepiness, further underscoring the importance of accurate oxygenation assessment in sleep apnea diagnosis.

Conclusion

Accurately diagnosing sleep apnea is essential for determining the appropriate treatment and improving patient outcomes. Polysomnography (PSG) remains the gold standard for sleep apnea diagnosis due to its comprehensive monitoring of sleep architecture and respiratory events. However, for patients who may not require such in-depth testing or have difficulty accessing sleep labs, Home Sleep Apnea Testing (HSAT) and newer technologies like Peripheral Arterial Tonometry (PAT) offer valuable alternatives.

Each diagnostic method comes with its strengths and limitations, and the choice of test should be tailored to the patient's symptoms, risk factors, and overall health. In addition to identifying the presence of apneas and hypopneas, oxygenation measurements, including Oxygen Desaturation Index (ODI) and nadir oxygen saturation, play a crucial role in assessing the severity of sleep apnea and its long term health risks.

With the increasing availability of portable diagnostic tools and advances in technology, sleep apnea diagnosis is becoming more accessible and accurate, allowing for earlier intervention and better management of this widespread condition.

CHAPTER 4: DIAGNOSIS BASED ON SEVERITY

Introduction

Sleep apnea is not a one-size-fits-all disorder; its severity can range from mild to severe, each with distinct clinical implications and management strategies. The severity of sleep apnea is usually determined by the Apnea-Hypopnea Index (AHI), which counts the average number of apneas (complete pauses in breathing) and hypopneas (partial reductions in airflow) per hour of sleep. In addition to the AHI, other factors such as oxygen desaturation levels, sleep fragmentation, and daytime symptoms are considered to provide a more comprehensive assessment of the severity of the disorder.

The severity of sleep apnea has a direct impact on treatment decisions and the urgency with which those treatments are applied. It also correlates with the long-term risk of cardiovascular diseases, metabolic disorders, and cognitive impairments. In this chapter, we will examine the different degrees of sleep apnea—mild, moderate, and severe—and discuss their diagnostic criteria, associated symptoms, and consequences if left untreated. We will also explore the role of different diagnostic tools in assessing severity and the therapeutic strategies for each category.

Understanding the Apnea-Hypopnea Index (AHI)

The Apnea-Hypopnea Index (AHI) is the most commonly used measure to quantify the severity of sleep apnea. It is calculated as the average number of apneas and hypopneas that occur per hour of sleep during a sleep study, such as polysomnography (PSG) or home sleep apnea testing (HSAT). A higher AHI indicates more frequent interruptions in breathing during sleep, which leads to greater disruption of sleep architecture and more severe health consequences.

The AHI is classified as follows:

> Mild sleep apnea: AHI of 5–14 events per hour
>
> Moderate sleep apnea: AHI of 15–29 events per hour

Severe sleep apnea: AHI of 30 or more events per hour

While the AHI is a useful tool, it does not capture the entire clinical picture of sleep apnea severity. Other factors, such as the Oxygen Desaturation Index (ODI), the nadir oxygen saturation, and the degree of daytime impairment, provide additional insight into the disorder's impact on an individual's health and quality of life.

Mild Sleep Apnea

Definition: AHI of 5–14 Events/Hour

Mild sleep apnea is diagnosed when the AHI falls between 5 and 14 events per hour. While the breathing interruptions are relatively infrequent in mild sleep apnea compared to more severe forms of the disorder, they still disrupt normal sleep patterns and can contribute to daytime fatigue and other health issues over time. In mild sleep apnea, the apneas and hypopneas typically do not lead to severe oxygen desaturation, but they are enough to fragment sleep and reduce its restorative value.

Symptoms of Mild Sleep Apnea

The symptoms of mild sleep apnea may be subtle or easily attributed to other causes, such as stress or poor sleep hygiene. Common symptoms include:

Occasional snoring: Snoring is a hallmark of obstructive sleep apnea (OSA), but in mild cases, it may occur less frequently or only in certain sleep positions, such as lying on the back.

Daytime fatigue: Individuals with mild sleep apnea may not feel excessively sleepy during the day but may still experience low energy levels, difficulty focusing, or a general sense of fatigue.

Mild morning headaches: Some individuals with mild sleep apnea wake up with headaches due to intermittent drops in oxygen levels during the night.

Restless sleep: Even though they may not wake up fully, patients with mild sleep apnea often experience restless or fragmented sleep, which can leave them feeling unrefreshed in the morning.

Mild mood disturbances: Irritability, anxiety, or mild depression can occur due to the disruption of normal sleep patterns.

Diagnostic Signs in Mild Sleep Apnea

In addition to an AHI of 5–14 events per hour, several other factors are considered when diagnosing mild sleep apnea, particularly in cases where the AHI alone may not capture the full extent of the disorder:

Minimal oxygen desaturation: Oxygen levels generally remain within the 90% or higher range in mild sleep apnea. The nadir oxygen saturation (the lowest oxygen level during the night) may dip slightly below 90%, but severe desaturation is uncommon.

Low Oxygen Desaturation Index (ODI): The ODI, which measures the frequency of oxygen desaturations of 3-4% or more, is typically low in mild sleep apnea, reflecting infrequent and less severe drops in oxygen levels.

Mild sleep fragmentation: While the individual may not be aware of frequent awakenings, there may be evidence of micro-arousals (brief periods of wakefulness) that disrupt normal sleep architecture.

Consequences of Untreated Mild Sleep Apnea

Although mild sleep apnea is less likely to cause immediate or severe health problems, it should not be dismissed as insignificant. If left untreated, mild sleep apnea can gradually worsen over time and lead to more serious consequences, including:

Progression to moderate or severe sleep apnea: Over time, mild sleep apnea can worsen, especially if contributing factors such as weight gain or aging occur. As the disorder progresses, the risk of cardiovascular complications and other health problems increases.

Daytime sleepiness and cognitive impairment: Even in mild cases, the repeated interruptions in sleep can lead to daytime drowsiness, poor concentration, and impaired cognitive performance.

Increased risk of metabolic issues: While the risk is lower than in moderate or severe sleep apnea, untreated mild sleep apnea has been associated with insulin resistance and an increased risk of developing type 2 diabetes.

Cardiovascular strain: Chronic sleep fragmentation and intermittent hypoxia can place stress on the cardiovascular system, contributing to high blood pressure, arrhythmias, and elevated heart rate.

Urgency of Treatment for Mild Sleep Apnea

The treatment of mild sleep apnea is important, though the urgency is often considered moderate. In many cases, lifestyle modifications and conservative treatment approaches can be effective in managing the condition and preventing its progression. These may include:

Weight loss: For individuals who are overweight or obese, losing weight can significantly reduce the severity of sleep apnea.

Positional therapy: Some patients with mild OSA experience apneas primarily when sleeping on their back. Positional therapy, such as sleeping on the side or using devices to prevent back sleeping, can alleviate symptoms.

Avoidance of alcohol and sedatives: These substances relax the muscles of the upper airway, increasing the likelihood of airway collapse. Avoiding them, especially before bedtime, can improve symptoms.

Mandibular advancement devices (MADs): These oral appliances, which reposition the lower jaw to keep the airway open, can be effective for mild sleep apnea, particularly in individuals who cannot tolerate CPAP.

CPAP therapy: In some cases, Continuous Positive Airway Pressure (CPAP) therapy may be recommended even for mild cases of OSA, especially if symptoms persist despite lifestyle changes.

Moderate Sleep Apnea

Definition: AHI of 15–29 Events/Hour

Moderate sleep apnea is diagnosed when the AHI falls between 15 and 29 events per hour. In moderate sleep apnea, the breathing interruptions are more frequent, leading to greater disruptions in sleep and more significant drops in oxygen levels. Individuals with moderate sleep apnea are more likely to experience noticeable symptoms that affect their daily functioning, and the disorder begins to pose a greater risk to long-term health.

Symptoms of Moderate Sleep Apnea

The symptoms of moderate sleep apnea are generally more pronounced than those of mild sleep apnea. Common symptoms include:

Loud snoring: Snoring in moderate sleep apnea is often loud, persistent, and disruptive to bed partners.

Excessive daytime sleepiness: Individuals with moderate sleep apnea may feel unusually tired during the day, even after what seems like a full night's sleep. They may have difficulty staying awake during sedentary activities such as watching TV or reading.

Morning headaches: Headaches are more common in moderate sleep apnea due to the more frequent drops in oxygen levels throughout the night.

Frequent awakenings: Many individuals with moderate sleep apnea are aware of waking up multiple times during the night, often due to gasping, choking, or a sensation of breathlessness.

Cognitive difficulties: Memory problems, poor concentration, and difficulty focusing are more pronounced in moderate sleep apnea, likely due to chronic sleep disruption.

Mood disturbances: Irritability, anxiety, and even depression may occur, exacerbated by poor sleep quality and oxygen deprivation.

Diagnostic Signs in Moderate Sleep Apnea

In addition to an AHI of 15–29 events per hour, moderate sleep apnea is characterized by more significant disruptions in oxygenation and sleep architecture:

Moderate oxygen desaturation: Oxygen levels may drop to around 85-90% during apneas and hypopneas, and the nadir oxygen saturation is often below 85% in more severe episodes.

Higher Oxygen Desaturation Index (ODI): The ODI in moderate sleep apnea is typically higher than in mild cases, reflecting more frequent and pronounced drops in oxygen levels.

Increased sleep fragmentation: Moderate sleep apnea causes more frequent arousals and micro-arousals, leading to significant disruption of sleep cycles and reduced time spent in deeper stages of restorative sleep.

Consequences of Untreated Moderate Sleep Apnea

If left untreated, moderate sleep apnea poses a significant risk to health and quality of life. The consequences of untreated moderate sleep apnea include:

Increased cardiovascular risk: Moderate sleep apnea is associated with a higher risk of hypertension, heart disease, arrhythmias, and stroke. The intermittent hypoxia and repeated surges in blood pressure during apneas put strain on the cardiovascular system.

Impaired cognitive function: Moderate sleep apnea is linked to memory problems, difficulty concentrating, and slower reaction times, which can affect both professional and personal life. It also increases the risk of dementia in older adults.

Higher risk of accidents: Daytime sleepiness caused by moderate sleep apnea can lead to drowsy driving and workplace accidents, posing a danger to both the individual and others.

Metabolic consequences: Untreated moderate sleep apnea can contribute to insulin resistance, weight gain, and the development of type 2 diabetes. Sleep fragmentation disrupts hormonal regulation of appetite, leading to increased hunger and cravings for high-calorie foods.

Urgency of Treatment for Moderate Sleep Apnea

The urgency of treating moderate sleep apnea is considered high, as the risks of untreated moderate OSA are significant. Treatment typically involves a combination of lifestyle modifications and medical interventions:

CPAP therapy: Continuous Positive Airway Pressure (CPAP) therapy is the first-line treatment for moderate sleep apnea. CPAP maintains an open airway by delivering a constant stream of air through a mask worn during sleep. It is highly effective at reducing the AHI and improving sleep quality.

Bi-level Positive Airway Pressure (BiPAP): For patients who have difficulty tolerating the pressure from CPAP, BiPAP may be recommended. BiPAP delivers two levels of pressure: a higher one during inhalation and a lower one during exhalation, making it easier for patients to breathe out against the pressure.

Mandibular advancement devices (MADs): In some cases, oral appliances such as MADs may be used as an alternative to CPAP, especially for patients who cannot tolerate CPAP or have mild-to-moderate sleep apnea.

Weight loss and lifestyle changes: For individuals who are overweight, losing weight can reduce the severity of sleep apnea. Exercise, dietary changes, and avoiding alcohol and sedatives can also improve symptoms.

Positional therapy: In patients whose sleep apnea is worse when lying on their back, positional therapy may be recommended to encourage side sleeping.

Severe Sleep Apnea

Definition: AHI of 30 or More Events/Hour

Severe sleep apnea is diagnosed when the AHI is 30 or more events per hour. This means that breathing is interrupted at least 30 times per hour, or once every two minutes, on average. Severe sleep apnea has a profound impact on both sleep quality and overall health, and it poses the greatest risk for serious long-term complications.

Symptoms of Severe Sleep Apnea

Individuals with severe sleep apnea often experience more intense and frequent symptoms that significantly disrupt their daily lives:

Severe daytime sleepiness: Daytime fatigue is extreme in severe sleep apnea, making it difficult for individuals to stay awake and alert during the day. They may struggle to function at work, school, or while driving.

Loud, chronic snoring: Snoring is typically loud and continuous, often waking up bed partners and disrupting their sleep as well.

Choking or gasping during sleep: Bed partners may observe the individual stopping breathing, followed by loud gasping or choking as they resume breathing.

Frequent awakenings: Individuals with severe sleep apnea may wake up multiple times per night due to airway obstruction, often with a sensation of choking or breathlessness.

Morning headaches and dry mouth: Waking up with headaches and a dry mouth is common in severe sleep apnea, due to the lack of oxygen and mouth breathing during the night.

Cognitive and mood disturbances: Severe sleep apnea can lead to significant cognitive impairment, including memory loss, difficulty concentrating, and poor decision-making. Mood disturbances such as depression, irritability, and anxiety are also common.

Diagnostic Signs in Severe Sleep Apnea

In severe sleep apnea, the physiological effects of repeated apneas and hypopneas are more pronounced:

Severe oxygen desaturation: In severe sleep apnea, oxygen levels often drop below 85%, and in some cases, they may fall below 80% during apneas. The nadir oxygen saturation is typically much lower than in mild or moderate cases, reflecting more frequent and severe drops in oxygen levels.

Very high Oxygen Desaturation Index (ODI): The ODI is significantly elevated in severe sleep apnea, indicating frequent and pronounced episodes of oxygen desaturation during the night.

Extreme sleep fragmentation: Severe sleep apnea causes frequent arousals and micro-arousals, leading to extensive fragmentation of sleep. This severely disrupts the normal sleep cycle, reducing the time spent in restorative stages of sleep (such as deep sleep and REM sleep).

Consequences of Untreated Severe Sleep Apnea

Severe sleep apnea poses a high risk for life-threatening health complications if left untreated. The consequences of untreated severe sleep apnea include:

Cardiovascular disease: Severe sleep apnea is strongly linked to a higher risk of hypertension, heart attack, stroke, congestive heart failure, and sudden cardiac death. The repeated drops in oxygen levels and surges in blood pressure during apneas place significant strain on the heart and blood vessels.

Cognitive decline: Severe sleep apnea is associated with cognitive dysfunction and an increased risk of dementia, especially in older adults. Chronic sleep disruption and hypoxia can lead to brain damage and impairments in memory, attention, and executive function.

Diabetes and metabolic syndrome: Untreated severe sleep apnea increases the risk of developing type 2 diabetes, insulin resistance, and metabolic syndrome. Sleep disruption affects the regulation of blood sugar and appetite hormones, contributing to weight gain and worsening metabolic health.

Increased mortality: Studies have shown that individuals with untreated severe sleep apnea have a significantly higher risk of premature death compared to those without the disorder, particularly due to cardiovascular events and stroke.

Urgency of Treatment for Severe Sleep Apnea

The urgency of treating severe sleep apnea is very high, as the condition poses an immediate threat to health and well-being. Treatment must be initiated as soon as possible to reduce the risk of life-threatening complications. The primary treatment options for severe sleep apnea include:

CPAP therapy: Continuous Positive Airway Pressure (CPAP) therapy is the most effective treatment for severe sleep apnea. It prevents airway collapse during sleep by delivering a continuous stream of air through a mask, which keeps the airway open and reduces apneas and hypopneas.

BiPAP therapy: In cases where CPAP is difficult to tolerate, Bi-level Positive Airway Pressure (BiPAP) may be used. BiPAP delivers higher pressure during inhalation and lower pressure during exhalation, making it more comfortable for patients with high pressure needs.

Adaptive Servo-Ventilation (ASV): For patients with complex sleep apnea syndrome (CompSAS) or a combination of obstructive and central events, ASV may be recommended. ASV adjusts the pressure in real-time based on the patient's breathing patterns.

Surgical options: In severe cases where CPAP or BiPAP is not effective, surgery may be considered. Surgical options include uvulopalatopharyngoplasty (UPPP), which removes excess tissue from the throat, and maxillomandibular advancement (MMA), which repositions the jaw to enlarge the airway.

Weight loss: For individuals who are obese, significant weight loss can reduce the severity of sleep apnea. Bariatric surgery may be considered for patients with severe obesity and sleep apnea.

Hypoglossal nerve stimulation (Inspire therapy): This emerging treatment option involves implanting a device that stimulates the hypoglossal nerve to prevent airway collapse during sleep. It is typically used for patients with severe OSA who are unable to tolerate CPAP.

Conclusion

The severity of sleep apnea is a critical factor in determining both the urgency and the type of treatment required. From mild sleep apnea, which may be managed with lifestyle changes and positional therapy, to severe sleep apnea, which demands immediate and aggressive intervention, each level of severity presents unique challenges and health risks. Polysomnography (PSG) and Home Sleep Apnea Testing (HSAT) are valuable diagnostic tools that help clinicians assess the severity of sleep apnea and develop appropriate treatment plans. By addressing sleep apnea at each stage, it is possible to improve sleep quality, daytime functioning, and long-term health outcomes for affected individuals.

CHAPTER 5: CHALLENGES IN DIAGNOSING AND TREATING SLEEP APNEA

IN DIFFERENT BODY TYPES

Introduction

Sleep apnea, particularly obstructive sleep apnea (OSA), is a widespread sleep disorder with significant health consequences. However, the way it presents, and the challenges it creates in diagnosis and treatment, can vary dramatically depending on an individual's body type. Body type influences both the risk factors and mechanisms behind sleep apnea, as well as how the disorder manifests clinically.

Although obesity is the most well-recognized risk factor for OSA, thin individuals can also develop the disorder, often due to different anatomical or neurological issues. The airway dynamics, distribution of fat, and presence of other health conditions can significantly alter how sleep apnea develops and how it should be managed. In this chapter, we will explore the unique challenges faced by both obese and thin individuals in the diagnosis and treatment of sleep apnea, examining how body type affects the condition and the various approaches needed to address these challenges.

Impact of Body Type on Sleep Apnea

Sleep apnea is primarily classified into three types: Obstructive Sleep Apnea (OSA), Central Sleep Apnea (CSA), and Complex Sleep Apnea Syndrome (CompSAS). OSA, by far the most common, occurs when the upper airway becomes blocked during sleep, while CSA is caused by a failure in the brain's signaling to the respiratory muscles, and CompSAS involves a combination of both OSA and CSA characteristics.

Body type, particularly weight and fat distribution, plays a significant role in OSA, influencing the likelihood of developing the condition and its severity. Although obesity is a key factor in OSA development due to increased fat around the neck and airway, non-obese individuals can also develop sleep apnea, especially if they have certain anatomical or neuromuscular abnormalities.

Obesity and Sleep Apnea

Obesity is the most commonly recognized risk factor for OSA, with research consistently showing that people with a higher body mass index (BMI) have an increased risk of developing the condition. The Wisconsin Sleep Cohort Study revealed that a 10% increase in body weight could result in a six-fold increase in the risk of developing OSA. The physiological mechanisms that link obesity and sleep apnea are primarily related to how excess weight affects the airway and respiratory function:

Fat deposition in the neck: Obese individuals often accumulate fat around the neck and throat, which leads to a narrowing of the upper airway. This makes the airway more prone to collapse during sleep when the muscles naturally relax.

Reduced lung volume: Excess fat in the abdomen can restrict lung expansion, reducing the amount of space for the lungs to fully expand during sleep. This decreases functional residual capacity (the volume of air left in the lungs after exhalation), making airway collapse more likely.

Systemic inflammation: Obesity is associated with chronic low-grade inflammation, which can contribute to upper airway swelling and increase the likelihood of airway obstruction during sleep.

Obesity is also associated with other conditions that exacerbate sleep apnea, such as metabolic syndrome, hypertension, and type 2 diabetes. These conditions increase the overall risk for cardiovascular complications in patients with OSA.

Thin Individuals and Sleep Apnea

Although much less common, thin individuals can also develop OSA. In these cases, the underlying causes are usually related to anatomical abnormalities or neuromuscular factors that make the airway more susceptible to collapse, even without excess fat:

Craniofacial abnormalities: Structural issues like a narrow airway, retrognathia (recessed jaw), or a high-arched palate can reduce the airway space and make collapse more likely during sleep.

Reduced muscle tone: Thin individuals may have reduced muscle tone in the upper airway, particularly if they suffer from neuromuscular disorders or aging-related muscle loss.

Genetic predisposition: Some people inherit specific traits that make them more likely to experience airway collapse during sleep, such as a smaller upper airway, even if they have a normal body weight.

Central sleep apnea (CSA), which is more common in individuals with certain neurological conditions or heart failure, is also seen more frequently in thin individuals than in obese individuals. Because CSA involves a failure of the brain's respiratory centers to send proper signals to breathe, the mechanism is different from the physical airway obstruction seen in OSA, making CSA harder to detect and treat in this population.

Diagnosing Sleep Apnea in Obese Patients

For obese individuals, the presentation of OSA is often more pronounced and readily identifiable. However, several challenges arise during the diagnostic process, particularly in distinguishing the severity of the condition and identifying the comorbidities that might affect treatment.

Key Diagnostic Tools

Polysomnography (PSG), the gold standard for diagnosing sleep apnea, is critical for accurately determining the severity of OSA in obese individuals. PSG records multiple physiological parameters, including brain activity, oxygen levels, heart rate, and respiratory effort, allowing for a comprehensive assessment of the patient's sleep patterns and identifying both apneas and hypopneas.

For obese patients, PSG is especially important for detecting comorbid conditions, such as hypoventilation syndrome or nocturnal hypoxemia, both of which are more common in individuals with higher body weight. These conditions may exacerbate sleep apnea and increase the risk of complications, making early diagnosis essential.

Home Sleep Apnea Testing (HSAT) may also be used in patients with a high suspicion of moderate to severe OSA, especially when access to PSG is limited. However, HSAT does not provide as much detailed information as PSG and may underestimate the severity of sleep apnea in obese individuals, particularly when comorbid conditions are present.

Impact of Obesity on Sleep Apnea Diagnosis

Obese individuals with sleep apnea often experience more severe symptoms and greater health risks compared to their thinner counterparts. Key diagnostic factors in obese patients include:

Higher Apnea-Hypopnea Index (AHI): Obese individuals tend to have more frequent and prolonged apneas and hypopneas, leading to a higher AHI. A higher AHI is correlated with an increased risk of cardiovascular complications, such as hypertension, heart failure, and stroke.

Increased oxygen desaturation: Obesity can lead to more pronounced oxygen desaturation events during sleep, often measured using the Oxygen Desaturation Index (ODI). A higher ODI indicates more frequent and severe drops in blood oxygen levels, which are linked to a greater risk of metabolic disorders and cardiovascular disease.

Hypoventilation: Obesity hypoventilation syndrome (OHS) is a condition where excess weight impairs breathing, leading to high carbon dioxide levels (hypercapnia) and low oxygen levels (hypoxemia), particularly at night. OHS is commonly associated with severe OSA, and diagnosing it is crucial for proper treatment.

Diagnostic Challenges in Obese Patients

Despite the strong association between obesity and OSA, diagnosing sleep apnea in obese individuals is not without challenges:

Comorbidities: Obese individuals often have multiple health conditions that complicate sleep apnea diagnosis, such as heart disease, diabetes, and hypertension. These comorbidities can mask or exacerbate the symptoms of sleep apnea, making it difficult to isolate the effects of the disorder.

Obesity Hypoventilation Syndrome (OHS): Obese patients with OHS present with more complex symptoms, including daytime hypoventilation, which can lead to confusion between OHS and more severe OSA. Differentiating between OSA and OHS is essential because the treatment strategies for these two conditions may differ.

Positional sleep apnea: Some obese patients experience positional OSA, where apneas occur primarily when sleeping on their back. Identifying positional apnea requires a detailed sleep study that tracks changes in breathing patterns based on sleep position.

Diagnosing Sleep Apnea in Thin Individuals

For thin individuals, diagnosing sleep apnea presents unique challenges. Because they do not fit the typical profile of an OSA patient, their symptoms may be overlooked or misattributed to other conditions. Additionally, thin individuals may be more likely to develop central sleep apnea (CSA) or complex sleep apnea syndrome (CompSAS), both of which require more advanced diagnostic techniques to detect.

Key Diagnostic Tools

While polysomnography (PSG) is essential for diagnosing sleep apnea in thin individuals, it plays an even more crucial role in identifying central sleep apnea and upper airway resistance syndrome (UARS). PSG is the only diagnostic tool that can measure the respiratory effort needed to distinguish between obstructive apneas, where the airway is blocked, and central apneas, where breathing stops due to a lack of effort by the brain.

In addition to PSG, other diagnostic tools may be necessary for thin individuals with suspected central sleep apnea or complex sleep apnea:

Capnography: This test measures carbon dioxide levels in the blood, which can help detect hypoventilation and distinguish between obstructive and central events.

Cardiovascular assessment: For individuals with central sleep apnea, particularly those with underlying heart conditions, a cardiovascular assessment is often needed to identify conditions such as Cheyne-Stokes respiration, a form of periodic breathing commonly seen in heart failure patients.

Diagnostic Challenges in Thin Individuals

The challenges of diagnosing sleep apnea in thin individuals are largely related to the less typical presentation of the disorder in this population. Some of the key difficulties include:

Atypical symptoms: Thin individuals with sleep apnea may not experience the classic symptoms of loud snoring or excessive daytime sleepiness. Instead, they may report restless sleep, morning headaches, or mild cognitive impairment, which can lead clinicians to misdiagnose the condition as insomnia, chronic fatigue syndrome, or anxiety.

Subtle presentation of central sleep apnea: Central sleep apnea (CSA) often presents with less noticeable symptoms than OSA. Thin individuals with CSA may not have any observable airway obstruction, making it difficult for bed partners or healthcare providers to detect the condition without the help of advanced sleep studies.

Lack of comorbidities: Unlike obese individuals, thin patients may not have the comorbidities that often prompt a sleep apnea diagnosis, such as hypertension or metabolic syndrome. This lack of associated conditions can lead to a delay in diagnosis and treatment.

Treatment Approaches for Obese Patients with Sleep Apnea

For obese individuals with OSA, treatment focuses not only on managing the airway obstruction but also on addressing the underlying causes of obesity and the associated health risks. Weight management, alongside traditional treatments such as Continuous Positive Airway Pressure (CPAP), plays a central role in the treatment of sleep apnea in this population.

CPAP Therapy

CPAP therapy remains the first-line treatment for OSA in obese individuals, as it prevents airway collapse by providing a continuous stream of air through a mask worn during sleep. However, CPAP adherence can be challenging for obese patients due to several factors:

Mask discomfort: Obese patients often have unique facial structures that make it difficult to find a comfortable mask fit, leading to air leaks or pressure points that make CPAP difficult to tolerate.

High pressure requirements: Obese individuals may require higher CPAP pressures to keep their airway open due to the increased weight around their neck and airway. High pressures can cause discomfort and may lead to difficulty exhaling against the pressure.

Comorbid conditions: Obese patients with comorbid conditions such as OHS or heart failure may require more complex treatment approaches, such as BiPAP (bilevel positive airway pressure), which provides lower pressure during exhalation to make breathing easier.

Weight Management and Bariatric Surgery

For many obese individuals, weight loss is a key component of treating sleep apnea. Reducing body weight can significantly decrease the severity of OSA by reducing fat deposits around the airway and improving lung function. Weight loss interventions may include:

Diet and exercise programs: For individuals with mild to moderate obesity, lifestyle interventions, including changes to diet and increased physical activity, can help reduce the severity of OSA.

Bariatric surgery: For individuals with severe obesity, bariatric surgery (such as gastric bypass or sleeve gastrectomy) may be recommended. Studies have shown that bariatric surgery can significantly reduce the severity of OSA, with some patients experiencing complete resolution of their sleep apnea symptoms after significant weight loss.

Surgical Interventions

In cases where CPAP is not effective or well-tolerated, surgical interventions may be considered. For obese patients, uvulopalatopharyngoplasty (UPPP), tongue reduction, or maxillomandibular advancement (MMA) may be recommended to remove or reposition tissues that are obstructing the airway.

In some cases, hypoglossal nerve stimulation (Inspire therapy) may be used as a treatment for OSA in obese individuals who cannot tolerate CPAP. This involves implanting a device that stimulates the muscles that control the airway, preventing collapse during sleep.

Treatment Approaches for Thin Patients with Sleep Apnea

Treating sleep apnea in thin individuals often requires a more tailored approach, particularly for those with anatomical abnormalities or central sleep apnea. Weight loss is not a consideration in this population, so treatment focuses on addressing the underlying causes of the disorder and managing the airway obstruction or neurological factors involved.

CPAP and BiPAP Therapy

For thin individuals with OSA, CPAP therapy is typically the first-line treatment, just as it is for obese individuals. However, thin patients may have different needs when it comes to mask fitting and pressure settings. Because thin individuals often have smaller airways or anatomical abnormalities, they may require higher CPAP pressures to keep the airway open.

For individuals with central sleep apnea, BiPAP therapy or adaptive servo-ventilation (ASV) may be required. ASV adjusts pressure in real-time based on the patient's breathing patterns, making it effective for treating central apneas and preventing hypoventilation.

Oral Appliances and Positional Therapy

Mandibular advancement devices (MADs), which reposition the jaw to prevent airway collapse, may be used for thin individuals with mild to moderate OSA who cannot tolerate CPAP. These devices are particularly effective for patients with retrognathia or other anatomical issues that contribute to airway obstruction.

Positional therapy may also be recommended for thin individuals with positional OSA, where apneas occur primarily when the patient is sleeping on their back. Positional therapy involves using devices or pillows to encourage the patient to sleep on their side, where airway collapse is less likely.

Surgical Interventions

For thin individuals with significant anatomical abnormalities, surgery may be necessary to correct the underlying cause of the airway obstruction. Common surgical procedures for thin patients with OSA include:

Uvulopalatopharyngoplasty (UPPP): This procedure involves removing excess tissue from the throat and soft palate to enlarge the airway and reduce the likelihood of airway collapse during sleep.

Maxillomandibular advancement (MMA): MMA surgery repositions the upper and lower jaw to enlarge the airway. This procedure is often used for patients with retrognathia or other craniofacial abnormalities that contribute to airway obstruction.

Tongue reduction surgery: In cases where the tongue is contributing to airway collapse, tongue reduction surgery may be used to reduce the size of the tongue and prevent it from blocking the airway during sleep.

Managing Central Sleep Apnea

For thin individuals with central sleep apnea, treatment may focus on addressing the underlying neurological or cardiovascular causes of the disorder. In some cases, medications such as acetazolamide or theophylline may be prescribed to stimulate breathing and reduce the frequency of central apneas.

In patients with CSA related to heart failure, treating the heart condition can sometimes improve the symptoms of sleep apnea. For example, improving cardiac function through medication or surgery can reduce Cheyne-Stokes respiration and improve overall breathing patterns during sleep.

Conclusion

Diagnosing and treating sleep apnea in different body types presents unique challenges that require personalized approaches to care. Obese individuals are more likely to develop OSA due to the mechanical effects of excess fat on the airway, and treatment often focuses on managing airway obstruction through CPAP therapy, weight loss, and surgical interventions. For thin individuals, sleep apnea may result from anatomical abnormalities or central nervous system dysfunction, requiring a different set of diagnostic tools and treatment strategies, including BiPAP therapy, ASV, and, in some cases, surgery.

By understanding the specific challenges faced by obese and thin patients, clinicians can develop more effective treatment plans that address the underlying causes of the disorder and improve both sleep quality and overall health outcomes. As sleep apnea research continues to advance, more targeted therapies will likely emerge, further improving the ability to tailor treatment to each patient's unique needs.

CHAPTER 6: TREATMENT OF MILD SLEEP APNEA

Introduction

Mild sleep apnea, characterized by an Apnea-Hypopnea Index (AHI) of 5-14 events per hour, is a condition where individuals experience relatively infrequent pauses in breathing or shallow breathing episodes during sleep. While mild compared to moderate or severe sleep apnea, it still warrants attention due to its potential effects on sleep quality and overall health. Left untreated, mild sleep apnea can progress into more severe forms and lead to complications such as daytime fatigue, cognitive decline, and an increased risk of developing cardiovascular disease, diabetes, and hypertension.

This chapter will explore the different treatment options for individuals diagnosed with mild sleep apnea. These options range from lifestyle changes and positional therapy to the use of mandibular advancement devices (MADs) and, in some cases, Continuous Positive Airway Pressure (CPAP). Treatment for mild sleep apnea is often less aggressive than that for more severe forms of the disorder, but the ultimate goal is to improve sleep quality, prevent progression, and reduce the health risks associated with untreated sleep apnea.

First-Line Therapies for Mild Sleep Apnea

In cases of mild sleep apnea, the initial treatment approach often focuses on conservative, non-invasive interventions. These therapies are aimed at reducing the frequency of apnea events and improving overall sleep quality without the need for more complex or invasive treatments. The most commonly recommended first-line treatments for mild sleep apnea include lifestyle changes, positional therapy, and the use of oral appliances.

Lifestyle Changes: Weight Loss, Alcohol Avoidance, and Sleep Hygiene

One of the most effective ways to manage mild sleep apnea, particularly for individuals who are overweight or obese, is through weight loss. Excess weight, especially around the neck and upper airway, contributes to airway narrowing and increases the likelihood of airway collapse during sleep. Losing as little as 10% of body weight has been shown to significantly reduce the severity of obstructive sleep apnea (OSA) by decreasing the amount of fat tissue around the airway.

Weight Loss and Its Impact on Sleep Apnea

Obesity is a major risk factor for sleep apnea, and neck circumference is one of the strongest predictors of OSA severity. Excessive fat deposits around the neck and throat place additional pressure on the airway, making it more prone to collapse during sleep. In mild sleep apnea, even modest weight loss can make a substantial difference.

Mechanism: Weight loss reduces the fat tissue around the upper airway, making it less likely to collapse during sleep. This can help reduce the frequency of apneas and hypopneas.

Benefits: A reduction in AHI, improved oxygen saturation levels, and fewer interruptions in sleep. Weight loss also has the added benefit of reducing the risk of cardiovascular diseases, improving insulin sensitivity, and enhancing overall physical health.

While the relationship between weight and sleep apnea is more pronounced in individuals with moderate to severe OSA, weight loss remains a crucial component in managing mild sleep apnea, especially when combined with other treatment strategies.

Avoiding Alcohol and Sedatives

For individuals with mild sleep apnea, avoiding alcohol and sedative medications (such as sleeping pills or benzodiazepines) is an important lifestyle modification. Both alcohol and sedatives cause the muscles of the upper airway to relax, increasing the likelihood of airway collapse during sleep. By avoiding these substances, patients can reduce the frequency of apneas and hypopneas.

Alcohol: Consuming alcohol, particularly in the evening, can worsen sleep apnea by increasing the relaxation of the muscles in the throat and lengthening the periods of apnea. Additionally, alcohol consumption can suppress the arousal response, which normally causes the sleeper to wake up briefly to restore normal breathing, thus prolonging periods of oxygen deprivation.

Sedatives: These medications further depress the central nervous system, increasing the risk of airway collapse during sleep and potentially exacerbating mild sleep apnea. By avoiding sedatives, individuals may prevent the worsening of apnea events.

For those with mild sleep apnea, limiting alcohol intake and avoiding sedative medications can significantly improve sleep quality and reduce the frequency of apneas, especially if used in conjunction with other treatment methods.

Sleep Hygiene and Optimizing Sleep Patterns

Improving sleep hygiene is another important aspect of managing mild sleep apnea. Good sleep hygiene includes habits and practices that promote healthy sleep patterns and create a favorable environment for uninterrupted rest. Some key aspects of sleep hygiene include:

Maintaining a regular sleep schedule: Going to bed and waking up at the same time every day helps regulate the body's internal clock, leading to more consistent and restful sleep.

Creating a sleep-conducive environment: Keeping the bedroom cool, quiet, and dark can improve sleep quality and reduce the likelihood of sleep disturbances. Using earplugs or white noise machines to block out noise and blackout curtains to minimize light can help.

Avoiding caffeine and heavy meals before bedtime: Caffeine is a stimulant that can disrupt sleep, and large meals close to bedtime can cause discomfort, both of which interfere with sleep quality.

Establishing a relaxing pre-sleep routine: Engaging in relaxing activities before bed, such as reading or taking a warm bath, can promote relaxation and make it easier to fall asleep.

By optimizing sleep hygiene, individuals with mild sleep apnea can reduce sleep fragmentation and improve their overall sleep quality, which may help reduce daytime fatigue and other symptoms associated with the condition.

Positional Therapy: Adjusting Sleep Position to Improve Breathing

For many individuals with mild sleep apnea, the supine position (sleeping on the back) exacerbates apneas and hypopneas because it allows the tongue and soft tissues of the throat to collapse into the airway. Positional therapy aims to prevent individuals from sleeping on their backs and encourages them to adopt a side-sleeping position, which helps keep the airway open.

How Positional Therapy Works

Positional therapy is based on the observation that OSA severity often worsens when individuals sleep on their back, a phenomenon known as positional obstructive sleep apnea. In side-sleeping positions, gravity no longer pulls the tongue and soft tissues backward into the airway, making it less likely for the airway to become blocked.

There are several methods used to encourage patients to sleep on their side:

Positional devices: There are specially designed devices that can be worn around the waist or back to prevent individuals from rolling onto their back during sleep. These devices may consist of small pillows, straps, or vests with soft supports that make back-sleeping uncomfortable.

Tennis ball technique: This is a simple and inexpensive method in which a tennis ball is sewn into the back of a sleep shirt or placed in a pocket on the back of a specially designed shirt. When the individual attempts to roll onto their back, the discomfort from the tennis ball encourages them to return to a side-sleeping position.

Pillows: Using pillows to prop the body up on one side can help keep individuals in a side-sleeping position. Special body pillows or wedge pillows can be used to prevent rolling over during sleep.

Effectiveness of Positional Therapy for Mild Sleep Apnea

Positional therapy can be an effective treatment for individuals with positional OSA, especially when combined with other lifestyle changes. Studies have shown that positional therapy can significantly reduce the number of apneas and hypopneas in patients with mild to moderate OSA, improving oxygen saturation levels and reducing sleep disturbances.

However, positional therapy may not be effective for all patients, particularly those whose sleep apnea is non-positional (i.e., apneas occur regardless of sleeping position). For these individuals, other treatments, such as CPAP or oral appliances, may be required.

Mandibular Advancement Devices (MADs): Oral Appliances for Mild Sleep Apnea

Mandibular advancement devices (MADs) are oral appliances designed to treat mild to moderate sleep apnea by repositioning the lower jaw (mandible) forward, which helps keep the airway open during sleep. MADs are commonly used for individuals with mild sleep apnea who prefer a less invasive and more comfortable alternative to CPAP therapy.

How Mandibular Advancement Devices Work

MADs are custom-fitted devices that are worn in the mouth during sleep. They work by pushing the lower jaw slightly forward, which helps prevent the collapse of soft tissues at the back of the throat, including the tongue and soft palate. This forward displacement of the jaw increases the space in the airway, reducing the likelihood of obstruction during sleep.

There are several types of MADs available, including:

Boil-and-bite devices: These are over-the-counter MADs that can be customized by boiling the device and then biting down on it to create an impression of the teeth. While less expensive than custom-made devices, boil-and-bite MADs may not fit as well or be as effective.

Custom-fitted MADs: These devices are made by a dentist or orthodontist who takes an impression of the patient's teeth and creates a device tailored to their mouth. Custom-fitted MADs are typically more comfortable and effective than over-the-counter options.

Effectiveness of MADs in Treating Mild Sleep Apnea

Several studies have demonstrated that MADs are effective in reducing AHI and improving sleep quality in individuals with mild to moderate sleep apnea. They are particularly useful for patients who cannot tolerate CPAP therapy or for those who prefer a more portable, less cumbersome option.

AHI reduction: MADs have been shown to reduce AHI by approximately 50% in patients with mild to moderate OSA. For individuals with mild sleep apnea, this reduction is often sufficient to alleviate symptoms and prevent progression of the condition.

Improved daytime symptoms: MADs can reduce daytime fatigue, improve cognitive function, and enhance overall quality of life for individuals with mild sleep apnea by reducing the number of apneas and hypopneas during the night.

Advantages and Limitations of MADs

Advantages:

Non-invasive and comfortable: MADs are less intrusive than CPAP therapy and do not require the use of masks or machines, making them a more comfortable option for many individuals.

Portable and easy to use: MADs are small and portable, making them convenient for travel or use outside the home.

Effective for mild to moderate OSA: Studies have shown that MADs are particularly effective for patients with mild to moderate sleep apnea, offering significant symptom relief.

Limitations:

Jaw discomfort or pain: Some individuals may experience discomfort in the jaw or teeth after prolonged use of MADs, especially if the device is not properly fitted.

Less effective for severe OSA: While MADs are effective for mild to moderate sleep apnea, they may not provide adequate relief for individuals with severe OSA, who may require CPAP or other treatment options.

Potential for dental issues: Long-term use of MADs may lead to dental problems, such as tooth movement, changes in bite alignment, or temporomandibular joint (TMJ) discomfort.

CPAP Therapy for Mild Sleep Apnea

Continuous Positive Airway Pressure (CPAP) is the gold-standard treatment for moderate to severe OSA, but it can also be used in individuals with mild sleep apnea, particularly if other treatments are ineffective or if the patient has significant daytime symptoms. CPAP therapy involves wearing a mask connected to a machine that delivers a continuous stream of air to keep the airway open during sleep.

When Is CPAP Therapy Recommended for Mild Sleep Apnea?

CPAP is typically recommended for individuals with mild sleep apnea if they:

Have significant daytime sleepiness: If lifestyle changes and other non-invasive treatments do not improve excessive daytime fatigue or cognitive impairment, CPAP may be prescribed.

Experience frequent awakenings: Individuals who wake up multiple times during the night due to breathing interruptions may benefit from CPAP therapy to stabilize their breathing.

Have coexisting medical conditions: Patients with mild sleep apnea who also have comorbidities such as heart disease, hypertension, or diabetes may be advised to use CPAP therapy to reduce their risk of complications.

Do not respond to other treatments: If lifestyle modifications, positional therapy, and MADs do not sufficiently reduce AHI or improve symptoms, CPAP therapy may be necessary.

Benefits of CPAP Therapy for Mild Sleep Apnea

While CPAP is more commonly used for moderate and severe OSA, individuals with mild sleep apnea can also experience significant improvements in sleep quality and daytime functioning with CPAP therapy:

Reduction in AHI: CPAP effectively reduces the AHI in individuals with mild sleep apnea, helping to prevent airway collapse and stabilize breathing throughout the night.

Improved oxygenation: By maintaining an open airway, CPAP prevents drops in oxygen saturation levels, reducing the risk of hypoxemia and associated health problems.

Enhanced sleep quality: CPAP therapy helps individuals with mild sleep apnea achieve deeper, more restorative sleep by preventing frequent awakenings and sleep disruptions.

Challenges and Adherence to CPAP Therapy

Although CPAP therapy is highly effective, many individuals with mild sleep apnea may find it difficult to adhere to treatment due to discomfort, mask issues, or the inconvenience of using the device every night.

Mask discomfort: Some patients experience discomfort with the CPAP mask, including irritation, pressure sores, or air leaks. Ensuring a proper mask fit and choosing the right type of mask (nasal mask, nasal pillows, or full-face mask) can help alleviate these issues.

Feeling claustrophobic: The sensation of wearing a mask connected to a machine can be overwhelming for some individuals, leading to feelings of claustrophobia. Gradual acclimatization to the mask, starting with short periods of use while awake, can help patients adjust.

Noise and dryness: The noise of the CPAP machine or the sensation of dry air can cause discomfort for some users. Humidifiers and newer, quieter CPAP models can help address these issues.

To improve adherence to CPAP therapy, patient education, mask fitting clinics, and support groups can provide individuals with the resources and support they need to use the device effectively.

Risks of Delaying Treatment for Mild Sleep Apnea

Even though mild sleep apnea may not seem as urgent as moderate or severe cases, delaying treatment can have negative consequences for long-term health and well-being. Untreated mild sleep apnea can progressively worsen over time, especially if contributing factors such as weight gain, aging, or other medical conditions arise. Some potential risks of delaying treatment include:

Progression to more severe sleep apnea: Over time, untreated mild sleep apnea can worsen, leading to a higher AHI and more severe symptoms. This increases the risk of developing moderate or severe OSA, which comes with a greater likelihood of cardiovascular complications and other health problems.

Increased risk of cardiovascular disease: Even mild sleep apnea can increase the risk of developing hypertension, heart disease, and stroke, particularly if the condition is left untreated for years. The intermittent hypoxia and sleep fragmentation associated with OSA can place stress on the cardiovascular system.

Cognitive impairment: Untreated sleep apnea can impair cognitive function, memory, and concentration, affecting daily performance and quality of life. Over time, these impairments can contribute to a greater risk of developing neurodegenerative conditions such as Alzheimer's disease.

Daytime fatigue and reduced quality of life: Without treatment, individuals with mild sleep apnea may continue to experience daytime fatigue, irritability, and a reduced ability to concentrate. This can impact job performance, social relationships, and overall quality of life.

Conclusion

Mild sleep apnea, while less severe than other forms of the disorder, still poses significant risks if left untreated. By addressing mild sleep apnea early through lifestyle changes, positional therapy, mandibular advancement devices (MADs), and, in some cases, CPAP therapy, individuals can improve their sleep quality, reduce the frequency of apnea events, and lower their risk of developing more severe health problems.

The most effective treatment plans are individualized, taking into account the patient's unique symptoms, risk factors, and preferences. For many individuals with mild sleep apnea, non-invasive treatments such as weight loss, alcohol avoidance, and sleep position modification may be sufficient to control the disorder. However, for those with more persistent symptoms, oral appliances or CPAP therapy may be necessary to achieve optimal outcomes.

By taking action early, individuals with mild sleep apnea can prevent the progression of their condition, improve their quality of life, and reduce the risk of long-term complications.

CHAPTER 7: TREATMENT OF MODERATE SLEEP APNEA

Introduction

Moderate sleep apnea, defined by an Apnea-Hypopnea Index (AHI) of 15-29 events per hour, is characterized by frequent interruptions in breathing during sleep. These interruptions, or apneas and hypopneas, lead to sleep fragmentation, reduced oxygen levels, and significant daytime symptoms, including excessive sleepiness, cognitive impairment, and increased risk of cardiovascular and metabolic complications.

While the treatment of moderate sleep apnea is less urgent than that of severe sleep apnea, it is still critical. Untreated moderate sleep apnea can lead to progressive worsening of symptoms, impaired quality of life, and heightened risks for serious health conditions such as hypertension, diabetes, stroke, and heart disease. The treatment approaches for moderate sleep apnea include a combination of Positive Airway Pressure (PAP) therapies, oral appliances, lifestyle changes, and other interventions aimed at reducing the frequency of apneas and improving overall health.

In this chapter, we will explore the primary treatment options for moderate sleep apnea, focusing on PAP therapy, oral appliances, and non-PAP alternatives. We will also discuss the consequences of untreated moderate sleep apnea and the strategies used to improve adherence to therapy.

PAP Therapy as the Primary Treatment

Positive Airway Pressure (PAP) therapy is the first-line treatment for moderate sleep apnea. PAP devices work by delivering a continuous or bi-level stream of air through a mask, which keeps the airway open during sleep, preventing apneas and hypopneas. PAP therapy has been shown to significantly reduce AHI, improve sleep quality, and lower the risk of long-term complications associated with moderate sleep apnea. The two most common forms of PAP therapy are Continuous Positive Airway Pressure (CPAP) and Bi-level Positive Airway Pressure (BiPAP).

CPAP Therapy: The Gold Standard

Continuous Positive Airway Pressure (CPAP) is the most widely used and most effective treatment for moderate sleep apnea. CPAP devices deliver a constant stream of pressurized air through a mask worn over the nose, or both the nose and mouth. The pressurized air acts as a splint, keeping the airway open throughout the night and preventing collapse.

How CPAP Works

CPAP therapy functions by maintaining a continuous positive pressure within the airway, ensuring that the soft tissues of the throat do not collapse during sleep. For patients with obstructive sleep apnea (OSA), this prevents the apneas (complete airway blockages) and hypopneas (partial airway blockages) that disrupt sleep.

In addition to reducing apneas and hypopneas, CPAP improves oxygen saturation levels, decreases the frequency of arousals (brief awakenings due to breathing disturbances), and enhances the quality of both REM sleep and deep sleep.

Benefits of CPAP Therapy for Moderate Sleep Apnea

Significant reduction in AHI: CPAP is highly effective in reducing the number of apneas and hypopneas per hour, often bringing the AHI down to normal or near-normal levels. This reduces the overall burden of the disorder and prevents further complications.

Improved oxygenation: By preventing airway collapse, CPAP therapy helps maintain normal oxygen saturation levels during sleep, reducing the risk of hypoxemia (low oxygen levels) and its associated health risks.

Enhanced sleep quality: CPAP therapy leads to fewer sleep disturbances and more consolidated sleep, allowing individuals with moderate sleep apnea to achieve deeper, more restorative sleep.

Reduction in daytime sleepiness: Many patients report feeling significantly more awake and alert during the day after starting CPAP therapy, as the therapy prevents the repeated sleep disruptions that contribute to excessive daytime sleepiness.

Decreased cardiovascular risk: By treating the underlying causes of sleep apnea, CPAP therapy helps reduce the strain on the cardiovascular system, lowering the risk of hypertension, heart disease, and stroke.

Challenges with CPAP Therapy: Adherence Issues

Despite its proven effectiveness, adherence to CPAP therapy is a major challenge for many patients. Studies have shown that up to 30-50% of patients with sleep apnea discontinue CPAP therapy within the first year of treatment due to issues with comfort, mask fit, or perceived inconvenience. Common adherence challenges include:

Mask discomfort: The mask used with CPAP therapy can cause irritation, pressure sores, or discomfort, particularly if it does not fit properly. Some patients also find the sensation of air pressure blowing into their nose or mouth to be uncomfortable.

Dryness or nasal congestion: The continuous stream of air can cause dryness in the nose or throat, leading to discomfort and nasal congestion. Many CPAP devices include a humidifier to address this issue, but it remains a barrier for some patients.

Feeling of claustrophobia: Some individuals feel claustrophobic while wearing the CPAP mask, especially if it covers both the nose and mouth. This can make it difficult to fall asleep or stay asleep.

Noise: Although modern CPAP machines are quieter than older models, some patients may still find the noise of the machine disruptive to their sleep or the sleep of their bed partner.

Strategies to Improve CPAP Adherence

Improving adherence to CPAP therapy is crucial for the long-term management of moderate sleep apnea. Several strategies can help patients overcome the challenges associated with CPAP use:

Proper mask fitting: Ensuring a proper fit for the CPAP mask is essential to minimizing discomfort. Many patients benefit from trying different types of masks, such as nasal masks, nasal pillows, or full-face masks, to find the option that is most comfortable for them.

Gradual acclimatization: For individuals who find it difficult to adjust to CPAP therapy, a gradual acclimatization process may help. This involves wearing the CPAP mask for short periods during the day while awake, allowing the patient to become more comfortable with the sensation of the mask and the air pressure before using it overnight.

Heated humidification: Many CPAP machines offer a heated humidifier option that adds moisture to the air, reducing dryness and nasal congestion. Using a humidifier can make CPAP therapy more comfortable and improve adherence.

Pressure adjustments: Some patients find the fixed pressure of traditional CPAP machines to be uncomfortable, especially during exhalation. Auto-titrating CPAP (APAP) or BiPAP devices, which adjust the pressure based on the patient's breathing patterns, may be more comfortable and help improve adherence.

Education and support: Providing patients with education about the benefits of CPAP therapy and offering support through sleep clinics or CPAP adherence programs can improve long-term use. Involving bed partners in the process can also help increase adherence.

BiPAP Therapy: An Alternative for Patients Struggling with CPAP

For some patients, particularly those with moderate to severe OSA or individuals who find it difficult to tolerate CPAP, Bi-level Positive Airway Pressure (BiPAP) may be recommended as an alternative. Unlike CPAP, which provides a constant level of pressure, BiPAP delivers two levels of pressure: a higher pressure during inhalation (to keep the airway open) and a lower pressure during exhalation (to make breathing out easier).

How BiPAP Works

BiPAP machines use a more flexible pressure delivery system, which can be particularly helpful for patients who have difficulty exhaling against the higher pressure used in CPAP therapy. By lowering the pressure during exhalation, BiPAP therapy allows patients to breathe more comfortably and reduces the sensation of struggling to exhale.

Benefits of BiPAP Therapy

Improved comfort: Many patients find BiPAP therapy more comfortable than CPAP, particularly if they struggle with the sensation of exhaling against constant pressure.

Pressure customization: BiPAP devices allow for more personalized pressure settings, making them ideal for patients with higher pressure requirements or those with comorbid conditions like obesity hypoventilation syndrome (OHS) or chronic obstructive pulmonary disease (COPD).

Reduction in central apneas: In patients with complex sleep apnea syndrome (CompSAS), BiPAP may be more effective than CPAP at reducing both obstructive and central apneas by providing more flexible pressure support.

Challenges with BiPAP Therapy

While BiPAP offers greater flexibility and comfort, it still requires a mask and air pressure delivery system, which can present the same adherence challenges as CPAP therapy. Mask discomfort, dryness, and feelings of claustrophobia can still occur, although patients who find BiPAP more comfortable than CPAP are generally more likely to adhere to the treatment.

Non-PAP Alternatives for Moderate Sleep Apnea

For patients who are unable to tolerate PAP therapy or prefer less invasive treatment options, several non-PAP alternatives are available for treating moderate sleep apnea. These alternatives include oral appliances, positional therapy, and lifestyle modifications.

Mandibular Advancement Devices (MADs)

Mandibular advancement devices (MADs) are oral appliances that are designed to treat moderate sleep apnea by repositioning the lower jaw (mandible) forward during sleep. By advancing the jaw, MADs help to keep the airway open and prevent the collapse of soft tissues that cause obstructive apneas.

How MADs Work

MADs work by slightly advancing the lower jaw and tongue, increasing the space in the upper airway and preventing obstruction. These devices are custom-fitted by a dentist or orthodontist and are worn in the mouth during sleep. MADs are typically recommended for patients with mild to moderate OSA who are unable to tolerate PAP therapy or prefer a non-invasive treatment option.

Benefits of MADs

Comfort and convenience: MADs are generally more comfortable and less intrusive than PAP therapy. They do not require a mask or machine and are easy to transport, making them a good option for patients who travel frequently.

Effective for moderate OSA: Studies have shown that MADs can effectively reduce AHI and improve sleep quality in patients with mild to moderate OSA. They are particularly useful for patients who have positional OSA, where apneas occur mainly when the patient is sleeping on their back.

Reduced daytime sleepiness: Like PAP therapy, MADs can help reduce excessive daytime sleepiness by preventing airway obstruction during sleep.

Limitations of MADs

Less effective than PAP therapy for severe OSA: While MADs are effective for patients with moderate sleep apnea, they may not provide adequate relief for individuals with severe OSA, who typically require PAP therapy.

Potential for discomfort: Some patients may experience jaw discomfort, tooth movement, or temporomandibular joint (TMJ) pain after prolonged use of MADs. Regular follow-up with a dentist is necessary to ensure that the device is working correctly and that no long-term dental issues arise.

Variability in effectiveness: The effectiveness of MADs can vary depending on the patient's anatomy and the severity of their OSA. While some patients experience significant improvements, others may require additional treatment options.

Positional Therapy: Managing Positional OSA

Positional therapy is a treatment approach that is often used in patients with positional OSA, a form of the disorder where apneas occur primarily when the patient is sleeping on their back. Positional therapy aims to encourage patients to sleep on their side, which can help prevent airway obstruction and reduce apneas.

How Positional Therapy Works

When patients sleep on their back, gravity pulls the tongue and soft tissues of the throat backward, increasing the likelihood of airway collapse. By sleeping on their side, patients can reduce the risk of airway obstruction and improve airflow.

Several methods are used to encourage side-sleeping:

Positional devices: Special devices, such as backpacks, belts, or vests with built-in supports, can be worn during sleep to prevent patients from rolling onto their back. These devices make back-sleeping uncomfortable, encouraging the patient to remain in a side-sleeping position.

Pillow or wedge supports: Using pillows or wedge supports to prop the patient up on their side can also help maintain the side-sleeping position throughout the night.

Benefits of Positional Therapy

Non-invasive and easy to implement: Positional therapy is a simple and non-invasive treatment that does not require a mask or machine, making it a comfortable option for many patients.

Effective for positional OSA: Studies have shown that positional therapy can significantly reduce the number of apneas and hypopneas in patients with positional OSA, improving sleep quality and reducing symptoms.

Limitations of Positional Therapy

Less effective for non-positional OSA: Positional therapy is only effective for patients whose apneas are significantly worse when they sleep on their back. Patients with non-positional OSA may not benefit from this approach.

Adherence issues: Some patients find positional devices uncomfortable and may have difficulty adhering to the treatment. Additionally, it can take time for patients to become accustomed to sleeping in a side position.

Lifestyle Modifications: Weight Loss and Avoiding Sleep Disruptors

For patients with moderate sleep apnea, lifestyle modifications can play an important role in managing the condition, especially when combined with other treatments. Weight loss and avoiding substances that can exacerbate sleep apnea, such as alcohol and sedatives, are key components of lifestyle management.

Weight Loss

Excess body weight, particularly around the neck and upper airway, contributes to the collapse of the airway during sleep. Losing weight can reduce the severity of sleep apnea by decreasing the amount of fat tissue around the airway and improving overall respiratory function.

Alcohol and Sedative Avoidance

Alcohol and sedatives relax the muscles of the upper airway, making it more likely for the airway to collapse during sleep. Avoiding alcohol and sedatives can help prevent the worsening of apneas and improve sleep quality.

Consequences of Untreated Moderate Sleep Apnea

Moderate sleep apnea is associated with significant health risks if left untreated. The frequent apneas and hypopneas that occur during sleep lead to intermittent hypoxia (low oxygen levels) and repeated arousals, which can have a negative impact on both physical and mental health.

Increased Cardiovascular Risk

Untreated moderate sleep apnea is strongly linked to an increased risk of developing hypertension, heart disease, stroke, and arrhythmias. The intermittent hypoxia and surges in blood pressure that occur during apneas place strain on the cardiovascular system, leading to endothelial dysfunction, inflammation, and sympathetic nervous system activation.

Metabolic Consequences

Moderate sleep apnea is associated with an increased risk of developing type 2 diabetes and metabolic syndrome. Sleep fragmentation and hypoxia can disrupt glucose metabolism and lead to insulin resistance, contributing to weight gain and worsening metabolic health.

Cognitive Impairment and Daytime Sleepiness

The repeated disruptions in sleep caused by moderate sleep apnea can lead to cognitive decline, memory problems, and difficulty concentrating. Untreated sleep apnea is also a major cause of daytime sleepiness, which can impair performance at work or school and increase the risk of accidents, particularly motor vehicle accidents.

Conclusion

Moderate sleep apnea requires timely and effective treatment to prevent the progression of the disorder and reduce the risk of long-term health complications. PAP therapy, particularly CPAP and BiPAP, remains the gold standard for treating moderate sleep apnea, offering significant improvements in sleep quality, oxygenation, and overall health. For patients who are unable to tolerate PAP therapy, alternatives such as oral appliances, positional therapy, and lifestyle modifications provide valuable options for managing the condition.

By addressing moderate sleep apnea early and adhering to treatment, individuals can improve their quality of life, reduce the risk of cardiovascular and metabolic complications, and enhance overall daytime functioning. Continued research and innovations in sleep apnea treatment will likely lead to further advancements in managing moderate sleep apnea, improving outcomes for patients around the world.

CHAPTER 8: TREATMENT OF SEVERE SLEEP APNEA

Introduction

Severe sleep apnea, defined as having an Apnea-Hypopnea Index (AHI) of 30 or more events per hour, is the most serious form of sleep-disordered breathing. Individuals with severe sleep apnea experience frequent apneas (pauses in breathing) and hypopneas (partial blockages of airflow), resulting in significant oxygen desaturation and frequent arousals from sleep. This leads to poor sleep quality, daytime sleepiness, and increased risks of serious health problems such as hypertension, heart disease, stroke, diabetes, and even sudden death.

Because of the profound health risks associated with untreated severe sleep apnea, early and aggressive treatment is critical. Treatment options for severe sleep apnea include Positive Airway Pressure (PAP) therapies, surgical interventions, and, in some cases, adaptive devices or pharmacological therapies. The goal of treatment is to prevent airway obstruction, restore normal breathing during sleep, and reduce the long-term risk of cardiovascular and metabolic complications.

This chapter will explore the various treatment options for severe sleep apnea, including advanced PAP therapies, surgical procedures, and emerging therapies such as hypoglossal nerve stimulation. We will also examine the consequences of untreated severe sleep apnea and the challenges involved in treating this high-risk group.

Advanced PAP Therapies for Severe Sleep Apnea

Positive Airway Pressure (PAP) therapy remains the gold standard treatment for severe sleep apnea. For most patients, Continuous Positive Airway Pressure (CPAP) is the first-line therapy. However, for patients with severe OSA or those who struggle with CPAP, more advanced PAP therapies like BiPAP or Adaptive Servo-Ventilation (ASV) may be required.

CPAP for Severe Sleep Apnea

Continuous Positive Airway Pressure (CPAP) therapy is widely recognized as the most effective treatment for sleep apnea, including severe forms. CPAP works by delivering a continuous stream of air through a mask worn over the nose and/or mouth during sleep, which keeps the airway open and prevents apneas and hypopneas.

How CPAP Works in Severe Sleep Apnea

In patients with severe sleep apnea, the airway collapses frequently during sleep, causing repeated interruptions in breathing. CPAP therapy maintains positive airway pressure, which acts like a splint to hold the airway open. This prevents the soft tissues of the throat, such as the tongue and soft palate, from collapsing and obstructing the airway.

In addition to reducing apneas and hypopneas, CPAP therapy improves oxygen saturation levels, reduces the frequency of arousals, and helps restore normal sleep architecture. This leads to more restful, restorative sleep and a significant reduction in daytime symptoms.

Benefits of CPAP for Severe Sleep Apnea

Significant reduction in AHI: CPAP is highly effective at reducing the number of apneas and hypopneas per hour of sleep. For most patients with severe OSA, CPAP therapy can reduce the AHI to normal or near-normal levels.

Improved oxygenation: By preventing airway collapse, CPAP maintains normal oxygen levels throughout the night, reducing the risk of hypoxemia (low blood oxygen levels). This is particularly important in severe sleep apnea, where oxygen desaturation can be profound.

Better sleep quality: CPAP therapy helps prevent frequent awakenings and disruptions in sleep caused by apneas, leading to more consolidated and restorative sleep.

Reduction in cardiovascular risk: Severe sleep apnea is strongly associated with an increased risk of cardiovascular diseases, including hypertension, heart failure, and stroke. By treating the underlying cause of sleep apnea, CPAP therapy helps reduce these risks.

Challenges with CPAP in Severe Sleep Apnea

Despite its effectiveness, adherence to CPAP therapy is a common challenge, especially in patients with severe sleep apnea who may require higher pressure settings to keep their airways open. The higher the pressure, the more difficult it can be for patients to adjust to CPAP therapy.

Common challenges with CPAP include:

Mask discomfort: Patients may experience discomfort from the CPAP mask, particularly if the mask does not fit properly or causes pressure points. Some patients may also develop skin irritation or pressure sores from the mask.

Feeling of claustrophobia: Some patients report feeling claustrophobic or anxious while wearing the CPAP mask, which can make it difficult to fall asleep or stay asleep.

Noise: Although modern CPAP machines are relatively quiet, some patients or their bed partners may still find the noise of the machine disruptive.

Dryness and nasal congestion: The continuous flow of air from the CPAP machine can cause dryness in the nose and throat, leading to nasal congestion or irritation. Using a heated humidifier can help alleviate these symptoms, but they remain a barrier for some patients.

Improving Adherence to CPAP Therapy

For patients with severe sleep apnea, adherence to CPAP therapy is critical for preventing complications and improving quality of life. Several strategies can help improve adherence to CPAP therapy:

Mask fitting clinics: Proper mask fit is essential for comfort and effectiveness. Many sleep clinics offer mask fitting services to help patients find a mask that fits well and is comfortable to wear.

Gradual acclimatization: Some patients may benefit from gradually adjusting to CPAP therapy by wearing the mask for short periods while awake before using it overnight.

Use of humidifiers: Adding a heated humidifier to the CPAP machine can help prevent dryness and nasal congestion, improving overall comfort.

Education and support: Providing patients with education about the benefits of CPAP therapy and ongoing support through follow-up appointments or support groups can improve long-term adherence.

BiPAP Therapy for Severe Sleep Apnea

For patients with severe sleep apnea who cannot tolerate CPAP or require higher pressure settings, Bi-level Positive Airway Pressure (BiPAP) may be recommended. BiPAP delivers two levels of pressure: a higher pressure during inhalation to keep the airway open and a lower pressure during exhalation to make breathing more comfortable.

How BiPAP Works

Unlike CPAP, which delivers a constant pressure throughout the breathing cycle, BiPAP adjusts the pressure during inhalation and exhalation. The lower pressure during exhalation makes it easier for patients to breathe out against the machine, which can be particularly helpful for patients with severe OSA who need higher pressure settings or for those with comorbid conditions such as chronic obstructive pulmonary disease (COPD) or obesity hypoventilation syndrome (OHS).

Benefits of BiPAP Therapy

Improved comfort: Many patients find BiPAP therapy more comfortable than CPAP, particularly if they struggle with exhaling against a constant pressure.

Better for high-pressure needs: BiPAP can provide higher levels of pressure than standard CPAP, making it a better option for patients with severe sleep apnea who require more pressure to keep their airway open.

Personalized pressure settings: BiPAP machines can be programmed with different pressure settings for inhalation and exhalation, allowing for more customized treatment based on the patient's needs.

Challenges with BiPAP Therapy

While BiPAP therapy can be more comfortable than CPAP, it still requires the use of a mask and an air pressure delivery system, which can present similar adherence challenges. Mask discomfort, dryness, and feelings of claustrophobia can still occur, though patients who find BiPAP more comfortable are more likely to stick with the treatment.

Adaptive Servo-Ventilation (ASV): A Treatment for Complex Sleep Apnea

For some patients, particularly those with complex sleep apnea syndrome (CompSAS), Adaptive Servo-Ventilation (ASV) may be the most effective treatment. CompSAS occurs when patients treated for obstructive sleep apnea (OSA) with CPAP or BiPAP therapy develop central apneas (pauses in breathing caused by the brain failing to signal the muscles to breathe). ASV is designed to treat both obstructive and central apneas by adjusting the pressure dynamically throughout the night based on the patient's breathing patterns.

How ASV Works

ASV machines continuously monitor the patient's breathing patterns and adjust the pressure in real time to stabilize breathing. If the machine detects that the patient is not breathing normally (such as during a central apnea), it increases the pressure to support breathing. When the patient's breathing returns to normal, the machine reduces the pressure to a lower, more comfortable level.

Benefits of ASV Therapy

Effective for complex sleep apnea: ASV is particularly effective in treating patients with CompSAS, where both obstructive and central apneas occur. By adjusting the pressure in real time, ASV can prevent both types of apneas and improve sleep quality.

Improved comfort: Because ASV machines only increase pressure when needed, they can be more comfortable than traditional CPAP or BiPAP machines, which deliver constant or bi-level pressure throughout the night.

Challenges with ASV Therapy

ASV machines are more complex and expensive than standard CPAP or BiPAP machines, and not all patients may be eligible for ASV therapy. For example, ASV is not recommended for patients with severe heart failure due to the risk of worsening heart function. Additionally, ASV therapy still requires the use of a mask and air pressure delivery system, which can present the same adherence challenges as other PAP therapies.

Surgical Options for Severe Sleep Apnea

For patients with severe sleep apnea who are unable to tolerate PAP therapy or who do not achieve adequate relief from non-surgical treatments, surgical interventions may be considered. Surgical options for sleep apnea are aimed at reducing airway obstruction by removing excess tissue, repositioning the jaw, or stimulating the muscles that control the airway.

Uvulopalatopharyngoplasty (UPPP)

Uvulopalatopharyngoplasty (UPPP) is one of the most common surgical procedures used to treat severe OSA. UPPP involves removing excess tissue from the soft palate, uvula, and throat to widen the airway and reduce the risk of airway collapse during sleep.

How UPPP Works

During UPPP, the surgeon removes excess tissue from the soft palate and uvula, and in some cases, parts of the tonsils may also be removed. By removing these tissues, the airway is widened, making it less likely to collapse during sleep.

Benefits of UPPP

Permanent reduction in airway obstruction: UPPP can provide long-term relief from obstructive sleep apnea by physically reducing the tissue that causes airway collapse.

Improved sleep quality: Many patients experience significant improvements in sleep quality after UPPP, with fewer apneas and hypopneas and less daytime sleepiness.

Limitations and Risks of UPPP

Variable success rates: The success of UPPP depends on the patient's anatomy and the severity of their OSA. While some patients experience significant improvements, others may not achieve full relief from sleep apnea symptoms.

Potential for complications: As with any surgery, UPPP carries risks, including infection, bleeding, and changes in voice or swallowing. In some cases, the procedure may also lead to velopharyngeal insufficiency, where air escapes through the nose during speech.

Maxillomandibular Advancement (MMA)

For patients with severe sleep apnea caused by structural abnormalities of the jaw, such as a receded jaw or narrow airway, maxillomandibular advancement (MMA) may be recommended. MMA is a more invasive surgical procedure that involves repositioning the upper and lower jaw to create more space in the airway and prevent airway collapse.

How MMA Works

During MMA surgery, the surgeon cuts the upper and lower jaw and moves them forward. This creates more space in the airway and reduces the likelihood of airway obstruction. The bones are then fixed in their new positions using plates and screws.

Benefits of MMA

Highly effective for severe OSA: MMA has one of the highest success rates of any surgical procedure for sleep apnea, with studies showing significant reductions in AHI and improvements in sleep quality.

Permanent relief: Unlike PAP therapy, which must be used every night, MMA provides a permanent solution to airway obstruction by addressing the underlying structural issues.

Risks and Limitations of MMA

Invasive surgery: MMA is a major surgical procedure that requires a long recovery period and carries the risks associated with any major surgery, including infection, bleeding, and potential changes in facial appearance.

Lengthy recovery: Patients undergoing MMA surgery may require several weeks to recover fully and may experience temporary discomfort, swelling, and difficulty eating.

Hypoglossal Nerve Stimulation (Inspire Therapy)

Hypoglossal nerve stimulation is a newer, minimally invasive treatment for patients with moderate to severe OSA who are unable to tolerate PAP therapy. The Inspire therapy system involves implanting a device that stimulates the hypoglossal nerve, which controls the muscles of the tongue. By stimulating the hypoglossal nerve, the device prevents the tongue from collapsing into the airway during sleep, keeping the airway open.

How Hypoglossal Nerve Stimulation Works

The Inspire device is implanted under the skin of the chest during a minimally invasive surgical procedure. A small wire runs from the device to the hypoglossal nerve, and another wire is placed near the ribcage to monitor breathing. During sleep, the device detects when the patient is trying to breathe and sends a mild electrical stimulation to the hypoglossal nerve, causing the tongue muscles to contract and move forward, preventing airway obstruction.

Benefits of Hypoglossal Nerve Stimulation

Effective for patients who cannot tolerate PAP: Inspire therapy offers a non-PAP alternative for patients with severe sleep apnea who are unable to tolerate CPAP or BiPAP therapy.

Minimally invasive: The implantation of the Inspire device is a minimally invasive procedure, and most patients recover quickly with few complications.

Improved sleep quality: Studies have shown that hypoglossal nerve stimulation can significantly reduce AHI and improve sleep quality in patients with moderate to severe OSA.

Limitations and Risks of Hypoglossal Nerve Stimulation

Surgical procedure: While the Inspire therapy system is minimally invasive, it still requires surgery, which carries the risks of infection, bleeding, and device malfunction.

Not suitable for all patients: Hypoglossal nerve stimulation is not appropriate for patients with central sleep apnea or for those with significant structural abnormalities of the airway.

Consequences of Untreated Severe Sleep Apnea

Severe sleep apnea, if left untreated, poses serious risks to both physical and mental health. The frequent apneas and hypopneas that occur during sleep lead to intermittent hypoxia (low oxygen levels) and repeated sleep fragmentation, which have a profound impact on the body's systems.

Cardiovascular Complications

Severe sleep apnea is strongly linked to an increased risk of cardiovascular diseases, including hypertension, heart failure, arrhythmias, and stroke. The repeated surges in blood pressure that occur during apneas place significant strain on the heart and blood vessels, leading to long-term damage.

Hypertension: Untreated severe sleep apnea is a leading cause of secondary hypertension, where high blood pressure is directly caused by another condition. The frequent oxygen desaturations and arousals associated with severe sleep apnea trigger the release of stress hormones like adrenaline, which raise blood pressure.

Heart failure: Patients with severe OSA are at increased risk of developing heart failure, particularly if they also have other risk factors like obesity or diabetes. The constant strain on the heart from apneas and hypopneas weakens the heart muscle over time.

Stroke: The intermittent hypoxia caused by severe sleep apnea increases the risk of stroke by promoting inflammation and endothelial dysfunction, which leads to the formation of blood clots.

Metabolic and Endocrine Consequences

Severe sleep apnea is associated with an increased risk of developing metabolic disorders, including type 2 diabetes, insulin resistance, and metabolic syndrome. Sleep fragmentation and intermittent hypoxia disrupt the body's glucose metabolism and lead to hormonal imbalances that increase appetite, promote weight gain, and reduce insulin sensitivity.

Type 2 diabetes: Patients with untreated severe sleep apnea are at a significantly higher risk of developing type 2 diabetes. The chronic sleep deprivation and hypoxia associated with sleep apnea impair the body's ability to regulate blood sugar, leading to insulin resistance and, eventually, diabetes.

Weight gain: Severe sleep apnea is also associated with obesity, partly due to the disruption of hormones that regulate hunger and satiety. Patients with sleep apnea often experience increased levels of ghrelin (a hunger hormone) and decreased levels of leptin (a hormone that signals fullness), which can lead to overeating and weight gain.

Cognitive Impairment and Daytime Sleepiness

The repeated interruptions in sleep caused by severe sleep apnea can lead to cognitive impairment, memory loss, and difficulty concentrating. Over time, untreated sleep apnea can contribute to a greater risk of developing dementia and Alzheimer's disease.

Daytime sleepiness: Severe sleep apnea is a major cause of excessive daytime sleepiness, which can impair job performance, reduce quality of life, and increase the risk of motor vehicle accidents.

Mood disturbances: Patients with severe sleep apnea often experience depression, anxiety, and irritability due to the chronic sleep disruption and poor quality of life associated with the disorder.

Increased Mortality Risk

Untreated severe sleep apnea is associated with a significantly increased risk of premature death, particularly from cardiovascular events such as heart attacks and strokes. Studies have shown that patients with severe sleep apnea have a two- to threefold increased risk of death compared to individuals without the disorder.

Conclusion

Severe sleep apnea is a serious and potentially life-threatening condition that requires prompt and aggressive treatment to prevent long-term complications. PAP therapy, including CPAP, BiPAP, and ASV, remains the gold standard for treating severe sleep apnea, offering significant improvements in sleep quality, oxygenation, and overall health. For patients who are unable to tolerate PAP therapy or who have anatomical abnormalities that contribute to airway obstruction, surgical interventions such as UPPP, MMA, and hypoglossal nerve stimulation provide valuable alternatives.

Early and effective treatment of severe sleep apnea can reduce the risk of cardiovascular disease, improve daytime functioning, and enhance quality of life. By adhering to treatment and addressing the underlying causes of sleep apnea, patients with severe OSA can achieve better health outcomes and reduce the risk of life-threatening complications. As research into sleep apnea continues, new and innovative therapies will likely emerge, further improving the management of severe sleep apnea and offering hope to patients around the world.

CHAPTER 9: NEW AND EMERGING TREATMENT OPTIONS FOR SLEEP APNEA

Introduction

Sleep apnea, especially obstructive sleep apnea (OSA), has become one of the most prevalent sleep disorders worldwide, affecting millions of individuals. Traditional treatments, such as Continuous Positive Airway Pressure (CPAP), Bi-level Positive Airway Pressure (BiPAP), and various surgical options, have been the cornerstone of managing moderate to severe sleep apnea. These treatments, while effective, have limitations, particularly regarding patient adherence, comfort, and long-term success.

In recent years, there has been significant progress in developing new and emerging treatment options that aim to provide more personalized, effective, and comfortable alternatives for managing sleep apnea. These innovations include hypoglossal nerve stimulation, positional therapy devices, and the integration of artificial intelligence (AI) in diagnosing and managing the condition. Additionally, drug therapies are being explored, and advancements in minimally invasive surgeries provide promising alternatives for patients who cannot tolerate traditional PAP therapies.

This chapter will explore the most promising new and emerging treatment options for sleep apnea, focusing on their mechanisms, effectiveness, and potential for improving patient outcomes.

Hypoglossal Nerve Stimulation: A Promising Alternative

One of the most significant innovations in treating moderate to severe obstructive sleep apnea (OSA) is hypoglossal nerve stimulation (HGNS). Hypoglossal nerve stimulation offers an alternative for patients who struggle with CPAP or other positive airway pressure therapies.

How Hypoglossal Nerve Stimulation Works

The hypoglossal nerve controls the movement of the tongue and muscles in the upper airway. In patients with OSA, the muscles of the upper airway relax too much during sleep, causing the airway to collapse and block airflow. Hypoglossal nerve stimulation works by stimulating the hypoglossal nerve, which helps move the tongue forward and prevent airway collapse during sleep.

The Inspire therapy system, one of the most widely known devices, is implanted under the skin of the chest. A small wire runs from the device to the hypoglossal nerve in the neck. Another sensor is placed near the ribcage to monitor breathing patterns. When the device detects the patient is trying to breathe, it sends mild electrical pulses to the hypoglossal nerve, stimulating the muscles and keeping the airway open.

Benefits of Hypoglossal Nerve Stimulation

Alternative for CPAP-intolerant patients: Many patients find CPAP uncomfortable or difficult to tolerate due to mask issues, noise, or claustrophobia. HGNS offers a minimally invasive alternative for these individuals.

Effective in reducing AHI: Clinical trials have shown that hypoglossal nerve stimulation can significantly reduce the Apnea-Hypopnea Index (AHI) in patients with moderate to severe OSA.

Studies have reported a 50-70% reduction in AHI after using HGNS.

Improved quality of life: By reducing apneas and improving sleep quality, HGNS helps alleviate daytime sleepiness, improve cognitive function, and enhance overall quality of life.

Minimally invasive: Unlike more invasive surgical procedures, such as maxillomandibular advancement (MMA) or uvulopalatopharyngoplasty (UPPP), HGNS is a minimally invasive procedure with relatively short recovery times.

Limitations and Challenges

Cost: Hypoglossal nerve stimulation is relatively expensive compared to traditional treatments like CPAP. The cost of the device and surgery may not be covered by all insurance plans, limiting access for some patients.

Not suitable for all patients: HGNS is not appropriate for patients with central sleep apnea (CSA) or those with severe obesity (often measured by a BMI over 32). Additionally, individuals with significant structural abnormalities of the upper airway may not benefit from this treatment.

Surgical procedure: While minimally invasive, HGNS still requires surgery to implant the device. Like all surgeries, it carries risks, including infection, pain, and potential device malfunction.

Hypoglossal nerve stimulation represents a promising option for patients who have failed to benefit from CPAP or other traditional therapies. The ability to target the tongue muscles directly and prevent airway collapse makes this a particularly innovative solution for treating moderate to severe OSA.

Positional Therapy Devices: Managing Positional Sleep Apnea

For patients whose sleep apnea is positional—meaning that apneas occur more frequently when sleeping on their back—positional therapy has long been a treatment strategy. While traditional approaches like the "tennis ball technique" have been used to prevent patients from rolling onto their back during sleep, new positional therapy devices have been developed to improve the efficacy and comfort of this treatment.

How Positional Therapy Devices Work

Positional therapy devices are designed to encourage patients to sleep in a side position by making back-sleeping uncomfortable. These devices range from wearable belts to vibration-based sensors that alert patients when they roll onto their back. Some of the most advanced devices include wearable monitors that detect sleep position and use gentle vibrations to nudge the patient back to a side-sleeping position without waking them up fully.

Examples of Positional Therapy Devices

1. NightBalance Lunoa: This device is worn around the chest and uses gentle vibrations to prompt patients to change their position when they start sleeping on their back. It adjusts the intensity of the vibration based on how the patient responds, ensuring that the vibration is enough to encourage position change without causing full wakefulness.

2. Zzoma Positional Device: This belt-like device is worn around the upper torso and prevents patients from rolling onto their back by providing a physical barrier. It is comfortable to wear and easy to adjust, making it a popular choice for patients with positional sleep apnea.

Effectiveness of Positional Therapy Devices

Reduced apneas: Positional therapy devices have been shown to significantly reduce the number of apneas and hypopneas in patients with positional OSA. Studies indicate that for patients whose apneas are primarily positional, these devices can lead to a 50-80% reduction in AHI.

Non-invasive and easy to use: These devices are non-invasive and do not require the use of a mask or machine, making them an attractive option for patients who prefer a simpler treatment.

Improved comfort compared to traditional techniques: While older methods, such as sewing a tennis ball into a shirt, were uncomfortable, new positional therapy devices are designed to be worn comfortably throughout the night.

Limitations and Challenges

Limited effectiveness for non-positional OSA: Positional therapy is only effective for patients whose sleep apnea is significantly worse when sleeping on their back. Patients with non-positional OSA may not benefit from these devices.

Adherence issues: Some patients may find it difficult to adjust to wearing a positional therapy device, particularly if they are used to sleeping on their back. Adherence to treatment may be lower compared to CPAP or other therapies.

Future Directions

Artificial Intelligence in Sleep Apnea Diagnosis and Management

The integration of artificial intelligence (AI) in healthcare is rapidly transforming the way sleep disorders, including sleep apnea, are diagnosed and managed. AI technology offers the potential to improve diagnostic accuracy, personalize treatment plans, and enhance patient adherence through automated monitoring and feedback systems.

AI-Enhanced Sleep Studies

One of the most significant applications of AI in sleep apnea is its use in analyzing sleep study data. Traditionally, sleep studies, particularly polysomnography (PSG), require manual scoring by sleep technicians. AI algorithms can now analyze these studies more rapidly and accurately, detecting apneas, hypopneas, and other sleep disturbances without human intervention.

Automated scoring: AI-powered sleep studies can automate the scoring process, providing clinicians with real-time data on sleep architecture and breathing events. This reduces the workload for sleep technicians and increases the speed at which diagnoses are made.

Improved diagnostic accuracy: AI algorithms can identify subtle patterns in sleep data that might be missed by human scorers, improving the diagnostic accuracy for sleep apnea and other sleep disorders. AI can also reduce the potential for human error, leading to more consistent and reliable results.

Personalized Treatment Plans Using AI

AI can also be used to develop personalized treatment plans for patients with sleep apnea. By analyzing a patient's sleep data, comorbid conditions, and treatment history, AI algorithms can recommend the most effective treatments and suggest adjustments to therapy based on real-time monitoring.

Tailored PAP settings: AI can be used to adjust CPAP or BiPAP settings dynamically, ensuring that the pressure delivered to the patient is optimal based on their unique breathing patterns. This reduces the need for frequent manual titration and ensures more comfortable and effective therapy.

Adherence tracking and feedback: AI-powered devices can track patient adherence to CPAP or other therapies and provide real-time feedback on their usage. Some systems can even send alerts to clinicians or patients if adherence drops or if there are issues with the therapy, such as mask leaks or inadequate pressure settings.

AI in Home Sleep Apnea Testing (HSAT)

Home Sleep Apnea Testing (HSAT) is becoming more common, especially for patients with a high probability of sleep apnea. AI-enhanced portable sleep monitors offer the ability to perform accurate diagnostics in the comfort of the patient's home, making sleep apnea testing more accessible and convenient.

Wearable devices: AI-powered wearable devices can monitor breathing, oxygen saturation, and sleep position while the patient sleeps at home. These devices can detect apneas and hypopneas with high accuracy and provide a complete sleep report to clinicians.

Cost-effective diagnosis: AI-enabled HSAT can reduce the cost of sleep apnea diagnosis by eliminating the need for overnight stays in a sleep lab. This makes sleep studies more accessible to patients who might otherwise delay or avoid testing due to cost or inconvenience.

The use of AI in sleep apnea management is still evolving, but it holds promise for improving long-term outcomes through predictive modeling. In the future, AI could help predict which patients are at risk for sleep apnea progression or comorbid conditions and recommend interventions before complications arise.

Pharmacological Therapies: A New Frontier in Sleep Apnea Treatment

While medications are not currently a primary treatment for sleep apnea, ongoing research is exploring the potential of drug therapies to treat both obstructive and central sleep apnea. These therapies aim to reduce the collapsibility of the airway, improve muscle tone, and modulate respiratory control in patients with sleep apnea.

Current Research in Drug Therapies

Several classes of drugs are being studied for their potential to treat sleep apnea, including:

1. Carbonic anhydrase inhibitors: Drugs like acetazolamide are being explored for their ability to increase ventilation and reduce the frequency of apneas in patients with central sleep apnea (CSA). Acetazolamide stimulates breathing by increasing the body's sensitivity to carbon dioxide.

2. Serotonin receptor agonists: Serotonin plays a role in maintaining airway muscle tone during sleep. Drugs that target serotonin receptors may help reduce airway collapse in patients with obstructive sleep apnea. Preliminary studies on ondansetron (a serotonin receptor antagonist) have shown promise in reducing apneas by improving muscle tone in the upper airway.

3. Hypoglossal muscle activators: Experimental drugs are being developed to stimulate the muscles of the tongue and upper airway, preventing collapse during sleep. These drugs aim to provide a pharmacological alternative to hypoglossal nerve stimulation.

Benefits and Limitations of Pharmacological Treatments

Non-invasive option: Drug therapies, if proven effective, would offer a non-invasive treatment option for patients with sleep apnea, making them an attractive alternative for individuals who cannot tolerate CPAP or prefer to avoid surgery.

Targeted approach: Pharmacological treatments could be tailored to address the specific underlying mechanisms of each patient's sleep apnea, such as airway collapsibility or central respiratory control.

However, drug therapies for sleep apnea are still in the experimental stage, and much more research is needed to determine their effectiveness and safety. Additionally, some drugs may have side effects that limit their use, and they may not be effective for all patients.

Minimally Invasive Surgical Options

In addition to hypoglossal nerve stimulation, other minimally invasive surgical procedures are being developed as alternatives to more traditional surgeries like UPPP or MMA. These less invasive procedures aim to provide long-term relief from OSA with shorter recovery times and fewer risks.

Radiofrequency Ablation (RFA)

Radiofrequency ablation (RFA) is a minimally invasive procedure used to shrink the tissues of the soft palate and tongue, reducing their size and stiffness and preventing airway collapse during sleep. RFA uses radiofrequency energy to create controlled lesions in the tissues, causing them to shrink over time.

Benefits: RFA is performed under local anesthesia and involves minimal discomfort and recovery time. It is a relatively quick procedure that can be performed in an outpatient setting.

Effectiveness: Studies have shown that RFA can reduce the severity of OSA in select patients, particularly those with mild to moderate sleep apnea and tongue-related obstruction.

Soft Palate Implants (Pillar Procedure)

The Pillar Procedure involves the implantation of small, polyester rods into the soft palate to stiffen the tissues and reduce the likelihood of collapse during sleep. This procedure is minimally invasive and can be performed under local anesthesia.

Benefits: The Pillar Procedure is less invasive than traditional surgeries like UPPP and has a shorter recovery time. It is particularly effective for patients with mild to moderate OSA who have palatal obstruction.

Effectiveness: While not as effective as CPAP, soft palate implants can improve sleep quality and reduce snoring and apnea events in select patients.

Conclusion

The landscape of sleep apnea treatment is rapidly evolving, with new and emerging therapies offering hope for patients who have not found success with traditional treatments. Innovations like hypoglossal nerve stimulation, positional therapy devices, and the integration of artificial intelligence into sleep studies are reshaping how sleep apnea is diagnosed and managed. Additionally, the exploration of pharmacological treatments and minimally invasive surgical options provides promising alternatives for patients seeking more comfortable and effective solutions.

While many of these emerging treatments show great potential, further research and clinical trials are necessary to fully understand their long-term effectiveness, safety, and applicability to different patient populations. Nonetheless, these advances represent a significant step forward in the quest to improve patient outcomes, enhance treatment adherence, and reduce the global burden of sleep apnea.

CHAPTER 10: COMMON PROBLEMS IN TREATMENT OF SLEEP APNEA

Introduction

Sleep apnea, particularly obstructive sleep apnea (OSA), is a chronic condition that significantly impacts patients' health and quality of life. While effective treatment options such as Continuous Positive Airway Pressure (CPAP) and Bi-level Positive Airway Pressure (BiPAP) exist, many individuals experience challenges in adhering to and tolerating these treatments. These problems can lead to poor treatment outcomes and increased risk of comorbidities associated with untreated or inadequately treated sleep apnea, such as cardiovascular diseases, cognitive impairment, and metabolic disorders.

In this chapter, we will explore the most common problems in the treatment of sleep apnea. We will focus on issues related to adherence to PAP therapy, difficulties encountered with surgical treatments, and the impact of cost and insurance barriers. Understanding these problems and addressing them effectively is crucial for improving patient outcomes and ensuring long-term success in managing sleep apnea.

Adherence to PAP Therapy

PAP therapy is considered the gold standard treatment for obstructive sleep apnea (OSA). It involves the use of a machine that delivers a stream of pressurized air through a mask worn over the nose, or both the nose and mouth, to keep the airway open during sleep. Despite its effectiveness in reducing apnea-hypopnea index (AHI) and improving sleep quality, adherence to PAP therapy remains a significant challenge.

Common Issues with PAP Therapy

Several factors contribute to poor adherence to PAP therapy, including mask discomfort, claustrophobia, machine noise, and other side effects. These challenges can lead to early discontinuation of treatment or inconsistent use, reducing the effectiveness of the therapy.

1. Mask Discomfort and Fit Issues:

One of the most frequently reported issues with PAP therapy is mask discomfort. Ill-fitting masks can cause air leaks, pressure sores, and skin irritation, making it difficult for patients to sleep comfortably.

Some individuals experience nasal congestion or dryness due to the constant airflow, particularly if their PAP machine lacks a built-in humidifier.

Patients with facial hair, unique facial structures, or dental issues may find it difficult to get a secure and comfortable mask fit, further complicating adherence.

2. Feeling of Claustrophobia:

Wearing a mask, especially one that covers both the nose and mouth, can induce a sense of claustrophobia in some individuals. This feeling can trigger anxiety, making it difficult for patients to relax and fall asleep while using PAP therapy.

Patients may experience panic attacks or an overwhelming sensation of being unable to breathe, even when the machine is working correctly.

3. Air Pressure Intolerance:

Some patients struggle to adapt to the constant air pressure delivered by their PAP machine, particularly during exhalation. The pressure required to keep the airway open can feel too forceful for some individuals, making it difficult to breathe out against the airflow.

High pressure settings, often required for patients with more severe sleep apnea, can exacerbate discomfort, leading to non-compliance with treatment.

4. Noise and Sleep Disruptions:

Although modern PAP machines are quieter than their predecessors, some patients and their bed partners still find the noise disruptive to sleep. The sound of the machine, combined with the airflow noise from mask leaks, can disturb both the patient and their sleeping partner.

Sleep fragmentation caused by PAP therapy-related noise can lead to increased daytime fatigue and dissatisfaction with treatment.

Strategies for Improving Adherence

Improving adherence to PAP therapy is critical for ensuring that patients receive the full benefits of treatment. Several strategies can help address the common issues that lead to poor compliance:

1. Proper Mask Fitting and Choice:

Personalized mask fitting is essential to ensure comfort and effectiveness. Sleep specialists should work closely with patients to find the most suitable mask type—whether it's a nasal mask, nasal pillows, or a full-face mask—that fits securely without causing discomfort.

Offering a variety of mask options, including nasal pillows for patients who dislike full-face masks, can improve comfort and adherence.

Mask-fitting clinics or trials with different mask models allow patients to try multiple options before committing to a specific mask.

2. Heated Humidification:

Adding a heated humidifier to the PAP machine can help alleviate dryness and nasal irritation caused by the airflow. Humidifiers add moisture to the air delivered by the PAP machine, reducing irritation and improving comfort.

Adjusting the humidification settings can also help patients who experience nasal congestion or dry throat due to dry air from the machine.

3. Pressure Adjustments and Auto-Titrating PAP:

For patients who have difficulty tolerating fixed pressure settings, auto-titrating PAP (APAP) machines can be an effective solution. APAP machines adjust the pressure throughout the night based on the patient's breathing patterns, providing higher pressure when needed and reducing it during more stable breathing periods.

BiPAP (bi-level positive airway pressure) machines can be beneficial for patients who struggle with exhaling against the high pressure of CPAP. BiPAP provides two different pressure levels—one for inhalation and a lower one for exhalation—making it easier to breathe.

4. Gradual Acclimatization:

Gradual acclimatization to PAP therapy, also known as desensitization, can help patients become more comfortable with the equipment over time. Patients may begin by wearing the mask for short periods while awake and gradually increase usage until they can sleep with the mask for the entire night.

Supportive coaching and education about the importance of long-term adherence can help patients overcome initial discomfort and anxiety.

5. Patient Education and Support:

Providing patients with comprehensive education about sleep apnea and the benefits of PAP therapy is essential for improving adherence. Patients need to understand how PAP therapy works, why it's necessary, and how it will improve their overall health.

Follow-up support from sleep specialists, including regular check-ins and encouragement, can improve long-term compliance. Peer support groups and online forums for sleep apnea patients can also provide valuable encouragement and shared experiences.

Surgical Challenges: Variability in Outcomes and Complications

For patients who cannot tolerate PAP therapy or do not achieve adequate relief from non-invasive treatments, surgical interventions may be considered. However, surgery for sleep apnea carries inherent challenges, including variability in outcomes, potential complications, and postoperative recovery issues.

Common Surgical Procedures for Sleep Apnea

1. Uvulopalatopharyngoplasty (UPPP):

UPPP is one of the most common surgical treatments for OSA. It involves removing excess tissue from the soft palate, uvula, and pharynx to widen the airway and reduce the risk of airway collapse during sleep.

2. Maxillomandibular Advancement (MMA):

MMA is a more invasive procedure that repositions the upper and lower jaw to increase the space in the airway and reduce obstructions.

3. Genioglossus Advancement (GA):

GA involves advancing the genioglossus muscle (the muscle that attaches the tongue to the lower jaw) to prevent the tongue from collapsing backward during sleep.

4. Hypoglossal Nerve Stimulation (HGNS):

HGNS, a newer and less invasive option, involves implanting a device that stimulates the hypoglossal nerve to prevent the tongue from obstructing the airway.

Challenges in Surgical Treatment

Surgical treatment for sleep apnea, while beneficial for some patients, presents several challenges that can affect both the immediate and long-term outcomes.

1. Variability in Outcomes:

Success rates for sleep apnea surgeries vary significantly depending on the procedure, the patient's anatomy, and the severity of the condition. For example, UPPP has a 50-60% success rate, with some patients achieving significant improvement, while others see minimal change in AHI.

Patient selection is crucial for surgical success. Patients with severe anatomical obstructions, such as those with small jaw structures or large tonsils, are more likely to benefit from surgery than those with more generalized airway collapsibility.

2. Postoperative Complications:

Like all surgeries, sleep apnea procedures carry risks of complications. UPPP can lead to painful swallowing, difficulty speaking, and changes in voice due to the removal of tissue in the throat.

MMA and GA, being more invasive, carry additional risks such as nerve damage, infection, bleeding, and jaw pain. These procedures require longer recovery times, and patients may experience difficulty eating or speaking during the healing process.

3. Long Recovery Times:

Surgical treatments for sleep apnea, particularly MMA and GA, can require several weeks or even months for full recovery. During this period, patients may experience pain, swelling, and temporary restrictions in their daily activities.

For patients undergoing hypoglossal nerve stimulation (HGNS), recovery is shorter, but patients still need time to adjust to the device and learn how to use the system effectively during sleep.

4. Inconsistent Long-Term Success:

While surgery may offer significant improvements in AHI and symptoms, some patients experience a recurrence of sleep apnea over time. Factors such as weight gain, aging, and changes in muscle tone can affect the long-term success of the procedure.

Patients must continue to monitor their sleep apnea and maintain lifestyle changes, such as weight management and avoiding alcohol, to preserve the benefits of surgery.

Insurance and Cost Barriers

The cost of treatment and insurance coverage can be significant barriers for patients seeking treatment for sleep apnea. Access to diagnostic testing, PAP therapy, and surgical interventions can be hindered by high costs, limited insurance coverage, and out-of-pocket expenses.

Insurance Coverage for Sleep Apnea Treatment

1. Coverage for Diagnostic Testing:

Most insurance plans cover polysomnography (PSG), the gold standard diagnostic test for sleep apnea. However, patients may face high co-payments or deductibles, which can deter them from seeking a diagnosis.

Home Sleep Apnea Testing (HSAT) is often covered as a lower-cost alternative to PSG, but its use may be limited to patients with a high pre-test probability of OSA.

2. Coverage for PAP Therapy:

Insurance plans typically cover the cost of PAP devices, but coverage varies depending on the plan and the type of machine. Some plans require patients to undergo compliance checks to ensure they are using the machine regularly before approving long-term coverage.

Out-of-pocket costs for PAP machines, masks, and accessories can be high, especially for patients with high-deductible plans. Replacing parts such as masks and hoses, which need to be replaced periodically, adds to the financial burden.

3. Surgical Coverage:

Surgical treatments for sleep apnea are usually covered by insurance if they are deemed medically necessary. However, coverage varies based on the procedure and the patient's condition.

Patients may face pre-authorization requirements, which can delay treatment. Additionally, some insurance plans may deny coverage for newer procedures, such as hypoglossal nerve stimulation, considering them experimental or not fully proven.

Out-of-Pocket Costs

For many patients, the out-of-pocket costs associated with sleep apnea treatment can be prohibitive. These costs may include:

Co-payments and deductibles for sleep studies and medical appointments.

Equipment costs for PAP machines, masks, and accessories.

Surgical fees, including hospital stays and anesthesia may not be fully covered by insurance.

Strategies to Address Cost Barriers

1. Flexible Payment Plans:

Sleep centers and medical equipment providers may offer flexible payment plans for patients who cannot afford the full cost of treatment upfront.

These plans allow patients to pay for their treatment over time, reducing the financial burden.

2. Patient Assistance Programs:

Some manufacturers of PAP machines and accessories offer patient assistance programs that provide financial support or discounted equipment for individuals with low income or high medical expenses.

3. Insurance Appeals:

If an insurance company denies coverage for a necessary treatment, such as surgery or hypoglossal nerve stimulation, patients can appeal the decision with the support of their healthcare provider. Successful appeals often involve providing detailed medical evidence of the necessity of the treatment.

Conclusion

The treatment of sleep apnea, particularly obstructive sleep apnea (OSA), is often met with a range of challenges that can hinder patient adherence, surgical success, and access to care. PAP therapy, while highly effective, is plagued by issues of comfort, pressure intolerance, and mask-related discomfort, all of which can reduce patient compliance. Similarly, surgical interventions, though beneficial for some, come with risks of complications, inconsistent outcomes, and lengthy recovery times.

Addressing these common problems requires a multifaceted approach that includes personalized care, patient education, and support systems to improve adherence to therapy and enhance treatment success. Additionally, overcoming financial barriers through flexible payment plans, patient assistance programs, and insurance advocacy is essential for ensuring that patients have access to the treatments they need.

By recognizing and addressing the challenges associated with sleep apnea treatment, healthcare providers can help patients achieve better health outcomes, reduce the burden of comorbidities, and improve quality of life for individuals living with sleep apnea.

CHAPTER 11: THE FUTURE OF SLEEP APNEA MANAGEMENT

Introduction

Sleep apnea, especially obstructive sleep apnea (OSA), is a serious and prevalent sleep disorder affecting millions of individuals worldwide. Untreated, it leads to significant health complications, including cardiovascular disease, metabolic dysfunction, cognitive decline, and an increased risk of accidents due to excessive daytime sleepiness. Despite the existence of effective treatments such as Continuous Positive Airway Pressure (CPAP) therapy and surgical interventions, many patients face difficulties adhering to or tolerating these options. These challenges, combined with the growing recognition of sleep apnea's public health impact, underscore the need for innovative solutions to improve diagnosis, management, and treatment outcomes.

The future of sleep apnea management is marked by technological advancements, personalized medicine, and public health initiatives aimed at improving early detection, patient adherence, and treatment outcomes. This chapter explores emerging trends, including the role of wearable technologies, artificial intelligence (AI), and minimally invasive therapies, along with the potential impact of public health policies and personalized treatment plans on the landscape of sleep apnea management.

Trends in Diagnosis: Simplified Home Tests and Wearable Technology

One of the most significant trends in sleep apnea management is the shift toward simplified diagnostic methods, particularly with the development of home sleep apnea testing (HSAT) and wearable devices. These innovations make it easier for patients to undergo diagnostic evaluations in the comfort of their homes, reducing barriers to testing and facilitating earlier diagnosis.

Home Sleep Apnea Testing (HSAT)

HSAT has already become an important tool in diagnosing sleep apnea, particularly for individuals with a high probability of having moderate to severe OSA. HSAT devices allow patients to record their breathing patterns, oxygen saturation, heart rate, and other relevant metrics while sleeping at home, without the need for an overnight stay in a sleep laboratory.

HSATs are generally less complex than traditional polysomnography (PSG), the gold standard for sleep apnea diagnosis. However, the future of HSAT will see advancements that improve both the accuracy and accessibility of home-based testing, particularly as AI-driven algorithms become integrated into these devices.

Improvements in HSAT Technology

1. Enhanced Accuracy: Current HSAT devices are designed primarily to detect obstructive sleep apnea (OSA), but advances in sensor technology and AI-based analysis will make it easier to diagnose more complex forms of sleep-disordered breathing, including central sleep apnea (CSA) and complex sleep apnea syndrome (CompSAS).

2. User-Friendly Designs: The next generation of HSAT devices will likely be smaller, more comfortable, and easier to use. This will reduce

the likelihood of user errors during the test, improving diagnostic reliability. Future devices may be incorporated into everyday objects such as smartphone apps, watches, or sleep headbands.

3. AI-Driven Data Analysis: By incorporating AI into HSAT devices, physicians will be able to automatically analyze test results and receive detailed reports highlighting specific apnea events, hypopneas, and other sleep disturbances. AI algorithms will also be able to triage patients, identifying those who require more immediate intervention or further diagnostic testing.

Wearable Devices and Sleep Apnea Detection

The development of wearable technologies offers exciting possibilities for continuous sleep monitoring and the early detection of sleep apnea. Wearables, such as smartwatches, rings, and headbands, are already being used to track heart rate, blood oxygen levels, and movement patterns during sleep. The future will see these devices becoming even more sophisticated, with improved ability to detect apnea events and provide actionable health insights.

Advances in Wearable Sleep Apnea Technology

1. Continuous Monitoring: Unlike traditional sleep tests, which are performed over a single night, future wearable devices will offer continuous monitoring of sleep patterns over extended periods, allowing for a more comprehensive evaluation of sleep apnea severity and treatment effectiveness.

2. Integration with Healthcare Providers: Wearable devices will be integrated with cloud-based platforms that allow healthcare providers to remotely monitor patients' sleep data and adjust treatment plans accordingly. This will be particularly useful for individuals undergoing treatment, as physicians can monitor adherence to therapies like CPAP or adjust settings based on the data collected by wearables.

3. Proactive Health Interventions: Wearable devices will not only track sleep apnea events but will also integrate with broader health metrics (e.g., physical activity, diet, stress levels). This will allow healthcare providers to recommend lifestyle interventions that can reduce the severity of sleep apnea, such as weight management or stress reduction techniques.

Challenges and Considerations

While HSAT and wearable technologies hold great promise for improving the diagnosis of sleep apnea, they also present certain challenges. Data privacy concerns and the accuracy of consumer-grade devices must be carefully managed. Regulatory bodies, such as the FDA, will need to establish standards for the safety, efficacy, and accuracy of sleep apnea wearables to ensure they meet clinical standards.

Innovations in Treatment: Advancing PAP Technology

and Minimally Invasive Therapies

While PAP therapy remains the most effective treatment for moderate to severe OSA, many patients find it difficult to adhere to. The future of sleep apnea management will focus on developing more comfortable, personalized, and user-friendly PAP devices, as well as exploring minimally invasive treatments that can offer long-term relief from sleep apnea without the need for nightly equipment.

Advances in PAP Technology

Continuous Positive Airway Pressure (CPAP) and Bi-level Positive Airway Pressure (BiPAP) therapy have been highly successful in treating OSA, but many patients struggle with discomfort, mask issues, or feelings of claustrophobia. The next generation of PAP devices will address these concerns by offering more comfortable and adaptive technologies.

1. Auto-Titrating PAP (APAP): APAP devices automatically adjust air pressure based on the patient's breathing patterns, delivering higher pressure during apneic events and reducing pressure during normal breathing. Improved algorithms will make these devices more responsive and adaptable, reducing discomfort and improving adherence.

2. Nasal EPAP Devices: Expiratory Positive Airway Pressure (EPAP) devices use the patient's exhalation to generate pressure, eliminating the need for a CPAP machine. Nasal EPAP devices, such as Provent and other emerging technologies, offer a small, non-invasive alternative that patients wear only on their nostrils during sleep. These devices may become more advanced and widely used in the future.

3. Quieter, Portable PAP Devices: Future PAP machines will likely become smaller, quieter, and more portable, making them more convenient for travel and less intrusive at home. These improvements will enhance patient comfort and encourage better adherence to therapy.

Smart PAP Devices and AI Integration

Artificial intelligence (AI) will play an increasingly significant role in PAP therapy, with smart PAP devices capable of real-time adjustments and automated feedback.

1. Real-Time Adjustments: Smart PAP devices will be able to analyze the patient's breathing in real-time and make instant adjustments to pressure settings based on sleep stage, body position, and respiratory effort. This will optimize the treatment, ensuring maximum efficacy without causing discomfort.

2. Feedback and Monitoring: AI-enabled PAP devices will offer automated feedback to both patients and clinicians, providing data on treatment adherence, mask fit, and sleep quality. This will allow for proactive management, with clinicians able to intervene early if problems arise.

Minimally Invasive Therapies

For patients who cannot tolerate PAP therapy or prefer more permanent solutions, minimally invasive surgical options will become more popular. Procedures such as radiofrequency ablation and hypoglossal nerve stimulation are already gaining traction as alternatives to traditional surgeries like uvulopalatopharyngoplasty (UPPP).

1. Hypoglossal Nerve Stimulation (HGNS): HGNS devices like Inspire have shown promise in treating moderate to severe OSA by stimulating the hypoglossal nerve to prevent airway collapse. Future iterations of HGNS devices will likely become more compact, energy-efficient, and customizable, improving patient comfort and long-term outcomes.

2. Soft Palate and Tongue Procedures: Radiofrequency ablation (RFA) uses heat to shrink and tighten tissues in the soft palate and tongue, reducing obstruction in the airway. This procedure is minimally invasive and can be done in an outpatient setting with quick recovery times. As technology advances, RFA devices will become

more precise, leading to better outcomes with fewer side effects.

3. Pillar Procedure: The Pillar Procedure involves inserting small implants into the soft palate to stiffen it and prevent collapse during sleep. As materials and techniques improve, this procedure may become more widespread, offering patients a less invasive option than traditional surgery.

Personalized Medicine in Sleep Apnea Treatment

The future of sleep apnea management will increasingly focus on personalized medicine, where treatment plans are tailored to the individual based on genetics, anatomy, and lifestyle factors. Rather than a one-size-fits-all approach, personalized medicine will allow for more effective and targeted treatments.

1. Genomic Profiling: Advances in genomic medicine will allow clinicians to identify patients who are genetically predisposed to sleep apnea or certain forms of sleep apnea (e.g., OSA vs. CSA).

This could lead to early interventions and the development of more effective treatment strategies based on a patient's genetic profile.

2. Anatomical Customization: 3D imaging and computer-aided design (CAD) technologies will enable the creation of customized oral appliances and surgical treatments tailored specifically to each patient's anatomy. For example, mandibular advancement devices (MADs) could be custom-designed based on detailed 3D models of the patient's airway, maximizing comfort and efficacy.

3. Comorbidity Management: Personalized treatment plans will consider a patient's broader health profile, including comorbid conditions like obesity, hypertension, and diabetes. This holistic approach will integrate lifestyle interventions, pharmacological treatments, and surgical options to address both sleep apnea and related health concerns.

Innovations in Public Health and Healthcare Policy

Addressing sleep apnea as a public health concern is essential to improving early detection, access to treatment, and patient outcomes. Sleep apnea is linked to a range of serious health conditions, including cardiovascular disease, diabetes, and depression, making it a significant burden on healthcare systems. Future public health initiatives and healthcare policy changes will focus on raising awareness, improving screening, and ensuring equitable access to diagnosis and treatment.

Increased Awareness and Education Campaigns

Public health organizations will play a key role in raising awareness about sleep apnea's risks and the importance of early diagnosis and treatment. Education campaigns targeted at both healthcare providers and the general public can help ensure that more individuals are screened for sleep apnea and receive appropriate treatment.

1. Public Health Campaigns: National and global public health campaigns can raise awareness about the symptoms of sleep apnea (e.g., snoring, daytime sleepiness, morning headaches) and encourage individuals to seek testing if they are at risk. These campaigns will also emphasize the link between sleep apnea and serious health complications like heart disease and stroke.

2. Healthcare Provider Training: Sleep apnea is often underdiagnosed because many primary care providers do not routinely screen for it. Medical

training programs will increasingly incorporate sleep medicine education, ensuring that healthcare providers are better equipped to recognize the signs of sleep apnea and refer patients for testing.

Improved Screening and Early Detection

Early detection is critical for preventing the long-term complications of sleep apnea. Future screening programs will focus on high-risk populations, such as individuals with obesity, hypertension, diabetes, or chronic respiratory conditions.

1. Integration into Primary Care: Routine screening for sleep apnea may become a standard part of primary care visits, especially for individuals with known risk factors. Screening questionnaires, combined with AI-driven diagnostic tools, will allow for more widespread detection of sleep apnea.

2. Workplace and School-Based Screenings: Sleep apnea screening programs may also be introduced in workplaces and schools, particularly for industries where excessive daytime sleepiness poses safety risks, such as transportation and

construction. Early detection in younger populations could help prevent long-term health consequences.

Access and Affordability of Treatment

One of the greatest challenges in managing sleep apnea is ensuring that patients have access to affordable and effective treatment. In the future, healthcare policies will focus on expanding coverage for sleep apnea diagnosis and treatment, particularly for underserved populations.

1. Insurance Coverage Expansion: Expanding insurance coverage for sleep apnea treatments, including PAP devices, oral appliances, and surgical interventions, will help reduce out-of-pocket costs for patients. This may include government-funded programs that ensure all patients have access to the treatments they need.

2. Telemedicine and Remote Monitoring: Telemedicine will play a critical role in expanding access to sleep apnea care, particularly in rural or underserved areas. Remote monitoring of PAP therapy adherence and virtual consultations with sleep specialists will make it easier for patients to

receive ongoing care without needing to visit a sleep clinic in person.

3. Subsidized Programs for Low-Income Patients: Government and nonprofit organizations will continue to develop subsidized programs for low-income patients, ensuring that the cost of sleep apnea diagnosis and treatment is not a barrier to care. These programs may offer free or discounted PAP machines, oral appliances, and surgical procedures to eligible individuals.

Conclusion

The future of sleep apnea management will be defined by technological innovation, personalized treatment approaches, and public health initiatives aimed at increasing access to care. Wearable devices, home sleep tests, and AI-driven diagnostics will make it easier to identify and treat sleep apnea early, while minimally invasive therapies and advances in PAP technology will improve patient comfort and adherence. Additionally, public health policies will focus on raising awareness, expanding screening programs, and ensuring that all patients have access to effective and affordable treatment options.

By leveraging these innovations, the healthcare community can significantly improve outcomes for individuals with sleep apnea, reduce the burden of comorbidities, and enhance overall public health.

CONCLUSION

Sleep apnea, particularly obstructive sleep apnea (OSA), is a critical public health issue affecting millions of people worldwide. Characterized by repeated pauses in breathing during sleep, it can lead to significant health problems, including cardiovascular disease, diabetes, cognitive impairment, and daytime fatigue. Over the past few decades, the understanding of sleep apnea has grown tremendously, from its initial clinical descriptions to the development of positive airway pressure (PAP) therapies and a range of surgical and non-invasive treatment options.

This book has explored the history, types, diagnosis, and treatment of sleep apnea, with particular emphasis on the challenges of managing this complex disorder in diverse patient populations. While current therapies, including CPAP, BiPAP, and surgical interventions, offer effective management, significant barriers remain—primarily issues of patient adherence, the complexity of diagnosis, and the variability in treatment outcomes. As sleep apnea continues to grow in prevalence, innovative solutions are emerging to enhance the diagnosis and treatment of this condition, from wearable technology and artificial intelligence (AI) to minimally invasive surgeries and personalized medicine.

Recap of Key Points

1. Sleep Apnea as a Public Health Challenge:

Sleep apnea, particularly OSA, is more than just a sleep disorder. It has profound implications for public health due to its association with chronic conditions like hypertension, stroke, heart disease, and diabetes. Untreated sleep apnea significantly increases the risk of these conditions, making early detection and effective management essential.

Beyond physical health, sleep apnea also affects mental health, contributing to mood disorders, anxiety, and cognitive decline. Many individuals with untreated sleep apnea experience depression, irritability, and difficulty concentrating, which can have detrimental effects on personal and professional relationships.

2. Types of Sleep Apnea:

Sleep apnea is not a monolithic condition. It presents in various forms, including Obstructive Sleep Apnea (OSA), where the airway becomes blocked, Central Sleep Apnea (CSA), where the brain fails to signal proper breathing, and Complex Sleep Apnea Syndrome (CompSAS), a combination of both obstructive and central components. These variations present distinct diagnostic and treatment challenges.

OSA is by far the most common form and is often associated with obesity and aging, but central sleep apnea can be seen in conditions such as heart failure, highlighting the importance of distinguishing between the different types for accurate treatment.

3. Diagnosis and Severity:

The Apnea-Hypopnea Index (AHI) remains the gold standard for diagnosing and classifying the severity of sleep apnea, dividing it into mild, moderate, and severe categories. Polysomnography (PSG), conducted in a sleep lab, is the most comprehensive diagnostic test, but home sleep apnea testing (HSAT) offers a more accessible and less costly option for many patients.

Diagnosis is crucial not only to confirm the presence of sleep apnea but to understand its severity and underlying causes, which inform treatment strategies. Identifying comorbid conditions such as hypertension, diabetes, and cardiovascular disease is also vital for tailoring treatment approaches.

4. Challenges in Treatment:

Adherence to treatment, particularly PAP therapy, remains one of the biggest challenges in managing sleep apnea. Many patients struggle with mask discomfort, claustrophobia, or pressure intolerance, leading to poor compliance. This can negate the benefits of therapy and leave patients at higher risk for long-term complications.

Surgical interventions, while offering long-term solutions for some patients, come with variable success rates and risk of complications. Uvulopalatopharyngoplasty (UPPP), maxillomandibular advancement (MMA), and hypoglossal nerve stimulation (HGNS) are among the options for patients who cannot tolerate PAP therapy, but these procedures are not suitable for everyone and carry risks related to recovery and long-term effectiveness.

5. Emerging and Future Treatment Options:

The future of sleep apnea management is promising, with technological innovations paving the way for more personalized and comfortable treatment options. Hypoglossal nerve stimulation (HGNS), radiofrequency ablation (RFA), and soft palate implants offer minimally invasive alternatives to traditional surgeries.

Artificial intelligence (AI) and wearable technology are transforming the landscape of diagnosis and management. AI-driven analysis of sleep study data, automated PAP titration, and wearable sleep monitors that provide continuous feedback are making it easier to diagnose and manage sleep apnea in a home-based setting.

Personalized medicine is becoming a reality, with genomic profiling and customized oral appliances that tailor treatment to each patient's unique anatomy and physiology. This approach promises to improve patient outcomes by addressing the specific factors contributing to their sleep apnea.

6. Public Health and Policy Implications:

Sleep apnea's growing prevalence and its association with other chronic diseases call for public health initiatives that focus on early detection, awareness, and intervention. Workplace screenings, education campaigns, and routine screening in primary care settings are all crucial strategies to reduce the public health burden of sleep apnea.

Healthcare policies will need to evolve to ensure broader access to sleep apnea treatments, particularly for underserved populations. This includes expanding insurance coverage for diagnostic testing and PAP devices, as well as offering subsidies for surgical treatments and innovative therapies for low-income patients.

Call to Action

Sleep apnea is a highly treatable condition, but the key to improving outcomes lies in early detection, adherence to treatment, and holistic management of associated health risks. There is an urgent need for increased public awareness about the dangers of untreated sleep apnea and the benefits of early diagnosis and treatment. Many individuals with sleep apnea remain undiagnosed, and even among those who are diagnosed, many do not receive adequate treatment due to adherence issues, cost barriers, or limited access to care.

Healthcare providers must continue to engage in patient education to ensure that individuals understand the importance of sleep apnea treatment and its impact on long-term health. Addressing the challenges related to treatment adherence—particularly in PAP therapy—will require innovative solutions, including personalized therapy plans, mask-fitting services, and ongoing support from sleep specialists.

Policymakers and public health organizations have a role to play in ensuring that screening for sleep apnea becomes a routine part of healthcare, particularly for high-risk populations. Subsidized programs and insurance coverage expansions will be essential for ensuring that all individuals have access to diagnostic testing and effective treatments, regardless of their financial situation.

Finally, research and development must continue to focus on improving the comfort, accessibility, and efficacy of treatments for sleep apnea. Technological innovations in wearable devices, AI-driven diagnostics, and minimally invasive therapies hold great promise for the future, but more research is needed to validate these new approaches and ensure that they meet the needs of diverse patient populations.

Looking Ahead: A Brighter Future for Sleep Apnea Management

As the understanding of sleep apnea deepens and treatment options expand, there is great optimism for the future. Technological advancements, coupled with a growing emphasis on personalized care, are transforming the way sleep apnea is diagnosed and managed. The integration of wearable technologies, AI, and minimally invasive treatments is making it easier for patients to access care, adhere to treatment, and achieve better outcomes.

Moreover, the focus on public health awareness and policy changes promises to reduce the burden of undiagnosed and untreated sleep apnea. By ensuring that sleep apnea is detected and treated early, we can prevent many of the serious health complications associated with this condition and improve the quality of life for millions of people around the world.

The future of sleep apnea management is bright, with new and emerging therapies offering hope for more effective, comfortable, and accessible treatments. As we move forward, it will be crucial to continue supporting research, improving healthcare policies, and engaging with patients to ensure that they receive the care they need to live healthier, more fulfilling lives.

By leveraging the power of technology, personalized medicine, and public health initiatives, we can look forward to a world where sleep apnea is not only manageable but where the quality of life for individuals living with the condition is significantly enhanced. Through collaboration between healthcare providers, policymakers, and patients, the future of sleep apnea management will undoubtedly lead to better health outcomes, improved patient experiences, and a reduced burden on healthcare systems globally.

D. A. Nyberg

BIBLIOGRAPHY

Books and Comprehensive Texts on Sleep Apnea and Sleep Medicine

Kryger, M. H., Roth, T., & Dement, W. C. (2016). Principles and Practice of Sleep Medicine (6th ed.). Philadelphia, PA: Elsevier.

> A foundational text covering all aspects of sleep medicine, including sleep apnea, diagnostics, and therapeutic options.

Guilleminault, C. (2001). Sleep Apnea Syndromes. New York, NY: Marcel Dekker.

> An in-depth exploration of sleep apnea syndromes, covering clinical presentations, diagnostic criteria, and treatment options.

Malhotra, A., & White, D. P. (2018). Obstructive Sleep Apnea. New York, NY: Springer.

> A detailed discussion of the pathophysiology, epidemiology, and

treatment of obstructive sleep apnea, including clinical guidelines and research updates.

Research Studies and Reviews on Sleep Apnea Prevalence and Impact

Peppard, P. E., Young, T., Barnet, J. H., Palta, M., Hagen, E. W., & Hla, K. M. (2013). "Increased prevalence of sleep-disordered breathing in adults." American Journal of Epidemiology, 177(9), 1006-1014.

> This study highlights the increasing prevalence of sleep apnea in the adult population and its associated risk factors.

Punjabi, N. M. (2008). "The epidemiology of adult obstructive sleep apnea." Proceedings of the American Thoracic Society, 5(2), 136-143.

> A review of the epidemiology of obstructive sleep apnea, covering prevalence, risk factors, and public health implications.

Diagnostic Methods and Sleep Study Research

Berry, R. B., Brooks, R., Gamaldo, C. E., Harding, S. M., Lloyd, R. M., Quan, S. F., & Troester, M. T. (2017). "The AASM manual for the scoring of sleep and associated events." Journal of Clinical Sleep Medicine, 13(4), 665-668.

> The American Academy of Sleep Medicine's scoring guidelines for polysomnography and sleep-related events, a key reference for sleep diagnostics.

Auckley, D. H., & Phillips, B. A. (2001). "Home sleep studies for obstructive sleep apnea." Respiratory Care Clinics of North America, 7(2), 351-364.

> Discusses the efficacy and reliability of home sleep apnea testing (HSAT) as an alternative to in-lab polysomnography for diagnosing obstructive sleep apnea.

Treatment and Management of Sleep Apnea

Sullivan, C. E., Issa, F. G., Berthon-Jones, M., & Eves, L. (1981). "Reversal of obstructive sleep apnea by continuous positive airway pressure applied through the nares." The Lancet, 317(8225), 862-865.

> A seminal study that introduced CPAP as an effective treatment for obstructive sleep apnea.

Grote, L., Hedner, J., Grunstein, R., & Kraiczi, H. (2001). "Therapeutic approaches to obstructive sleep apnea: Past, present, and future." Sleep Medicine Reviews, 5(5), 509-530.

> Reviews the evolution of sleep apnea treatments, including emerging therapies and the future directions of sleep medicine.

Gagnadoux, F., & Le Vaillant, M. (2021). "Hypoglossal nerve stimulation in obstructive sleep apnea: Systematic review and meta-analysis." European Respiratory Journal, 58(1), 2100022.

> A systematic review and meta-analysis on hypoglossal nerve stimulation, an emerging therapy for sleep apnea, with a focus on clinical outcomes and patient adherence.

Public Health and Policy Implications

Peppard, P. E., Young, T., Palta, M., & Skatrud, J. (2000). "Prospective study of the association between sleep-disordered breathing and hypertension." New England Journal of Medicine, 342(19), 1378-1384.

> This study examines the link between sleep apnea and hypertension, underscoring the public health significance of the disorder.

Strohl, K. P., & Brown, D. B. (2012). "Policy and public health perspectives on sleep disordered breathing." American Journal of Respiratory and Critical Care Medicine, 185(10), 1115-1122.

> Explores the public health implications of sleep apnea, focusing on screening, treatment access, and the economic burden of untreated sleep apnea.

Pack, A. I. (2016). "Sleep apnea and the public health challenge of sleep disorders." American Journal of Public Health, 106(9), 1572-1575.

> A discussion on the need for increased public health focus on sleep disorders and the importance of early detection and treatment.

Emerging Technologies and Future Directions

Tarasiuk, A., & Reuveni, H. (2013). "The economic impact of obstructive sleep apnea." Current Opinion in Pulmonary Medicine, 19(6), 639-644.

> Analyzes the economic impact of sleep apnea and the cost-effectiveness of new treatment technologies, including wearables and home sleep monitoring.

Kuna, S. T., Gurubhagavatula, I., Maislin, G., Hin, S., Hartwig, K. C., McCloskey, S., & Pack, A. I. (2011). "Non-inferiority of functional outcomes in home and laboratory polysomnography." Sleep, 34(4), 403-414.

> Compares outcomes between home-based and laboratory-based polysomnography, exploring future applications of home sleep monitoring technologies.

Mason, M., & Takahashi, S. (2018). "Artificial intelligence in sleep medicine: Revolutionizing diagnosis and treatment." Sleep Medicine Clinics, 13(4), 587-599.

> Examines the role of AI in sleep medicine, including advancements in diagnostic tools, PAP therapy customization, and patient monitoring.

Comprehensive Reviews on Sleep Apnea and Health

Redline, S., & Young, T. (2010). "Epidemiology and natural history of obstructive sleep apnea." Proceedings of the American Thoracic Society, 5(2), 119-126.

> A comprehensive review of the epidemiology, risk factors, and progression of sleep apnea, with a focus on public health implications.

McNicholas, W. T., & Bonsignore, M. R. (2007). "Sleep apnea as an independent risk factor for cardiovascular disease: Current evidence, basic mechanisms, and research priorities." European Respiratory Journal, 29(1), 156-178.

> Discusses the link between sleep apnea and cardiovascular disease, focusing on current research and future priorities for improving patient outcomes.

Iftikhar, I. H., Kline, C. E., Youngstedt, S. D., & Bogan, R. K. (2014). "Effects of exercise training on sleep apnea: A meta-analysis." Lung, 192(1), 175-184.

> A meta-analysis examining the effects of exercise as a non-invasive treatment option for sleep apnea, particularly useful for individuals seeking lifestyle-based interventions.

Patient and Clinical Guides

Epstein, L. J., Kristo, D., Strollo, P. J., Friedman, N., Malhotra, A., Patil, S. P., & Weinstein, M. D. (2009). "Clinical guideline for the evaluation, management and long-term care of obstructive sleep apnea in adults." Journal of Clinical Sleep Medicine, 5(3), 263-276.

> Provides guidelines for clinicians on managing sleep apnea, including diagnosis, treatment options, and long-term care strategies.

Kapur, V. K., Auckley, D. H., Chowdhuri, S., Kuhlmann, D. C., Mehra, R., Ramar, K., & Harrod,

C. G. (2017). "Clinical practice guideline for diagnostic testing for adult obstructive sleep apnea." Journal of Clinical Sleep Medicine, 13(3), 479-504.

> This guideline offers insights for healthcare professionals on diagnostic testing options for adult obstructive sleep apnea, including indications for home sleep testing.

*****

www.ingramcontent.com/pod-product-compliance
Lightning Source LLC
Chambersburg PA
CBHW052345220526

45465CB00003BA/967